TESTIMONIALS

"When we think of martial arts, especially reality-based, we must consider the subject matter as well as the audience, and how to deliver the information with an effective impact. When speaking of specialized topics such as real-world personal protection skills for women, few can deliver TRUTH-based information and technique like Sho-Dai Soke Mike Andrus.

Grand Master Andrus is one of the very few subject-matter experts on women's personal protection and has developed a program that is both effective and pragmatic.

In this book, one will find life-saving techniques and methodologies that I believe have revolutionized the science of women's personal protection.

A true master of his craft, Mr. Mike does not rely on theory and lip service . . . he can deliver on the mat or in the street! Anyone (man or woman) interested in an eye-opening lesson on what it takes to stay alive in today's often volatile urban landscape must read this book! I suggest that every parent make this book a mandatory read for their female children, and this book should be in the dorm room of every female university student worldwide!

Grand Master Andrus has done a superior job in the creation of this curriculum, and I urge you to take advantage of this information and arm yourself with the knowledge from one of the world's leading subject-matter experts on this topic."

Soke David D'Antonio
Ninjutsu (Wada-Ha Koga Ryu) 10th Dan
Scientific Martial Arts 9th Dan
C.U.T.S. Founder (Critical Urban Tactical Strategies)

"Master Mike Andrus' book is direct and to the point. It is effective and very easy to understand. Great for women of any age." *Sifu Cliff Kupper, 4th Generation Kung Fu Master of Ip Man*

"Mike is a very caring, proficient Martial Artist. He has great technical skills and a great teaching style. He truly is one of the great teachers, especially in the world of Women's Self-Defense." *Master Dana Kiklis, 4th Degree Black Belt*

"This workshop is so needed. As a woman, as a martial artist and as a martial arts instructor, I know this will be invaluable. Even if you have taken other self-defense classes, even if you teach them yourself, being able to take advantage of learning from another's perspective, especially someone with Sensei Mike's expertise, and being able to hone your own skills to stay fresh is so important. This is a fabulous opportunity for all women!" *Sijo Khadi Madama, The Iron Butterfly, Founder, Fa Shen Training Arts, 3 time Hall of Fame Award Inductee*

"Mike has been an asset to the restaurant's safety and has been a great advocate of ours." **The Freight House Cafe, LTD**

"Thank you so much for doing the presentation for the women's group...fabulous! You opened a lot of eyes...thanks again!" **Kelly Willey**

"Any women who miss this seminar are losing out. Master Mike is an amazing instructor and a well-respected associate of mine. He is also the GNPRBFI Women's Self Defense Instructor of the Year! Mike has the skills to teach you how to stay alive. HE HAS MY FULL BACKING AND SUPPORT!" **Soke D'Antonio, 10th Dan, C.U.T.S. Founder**

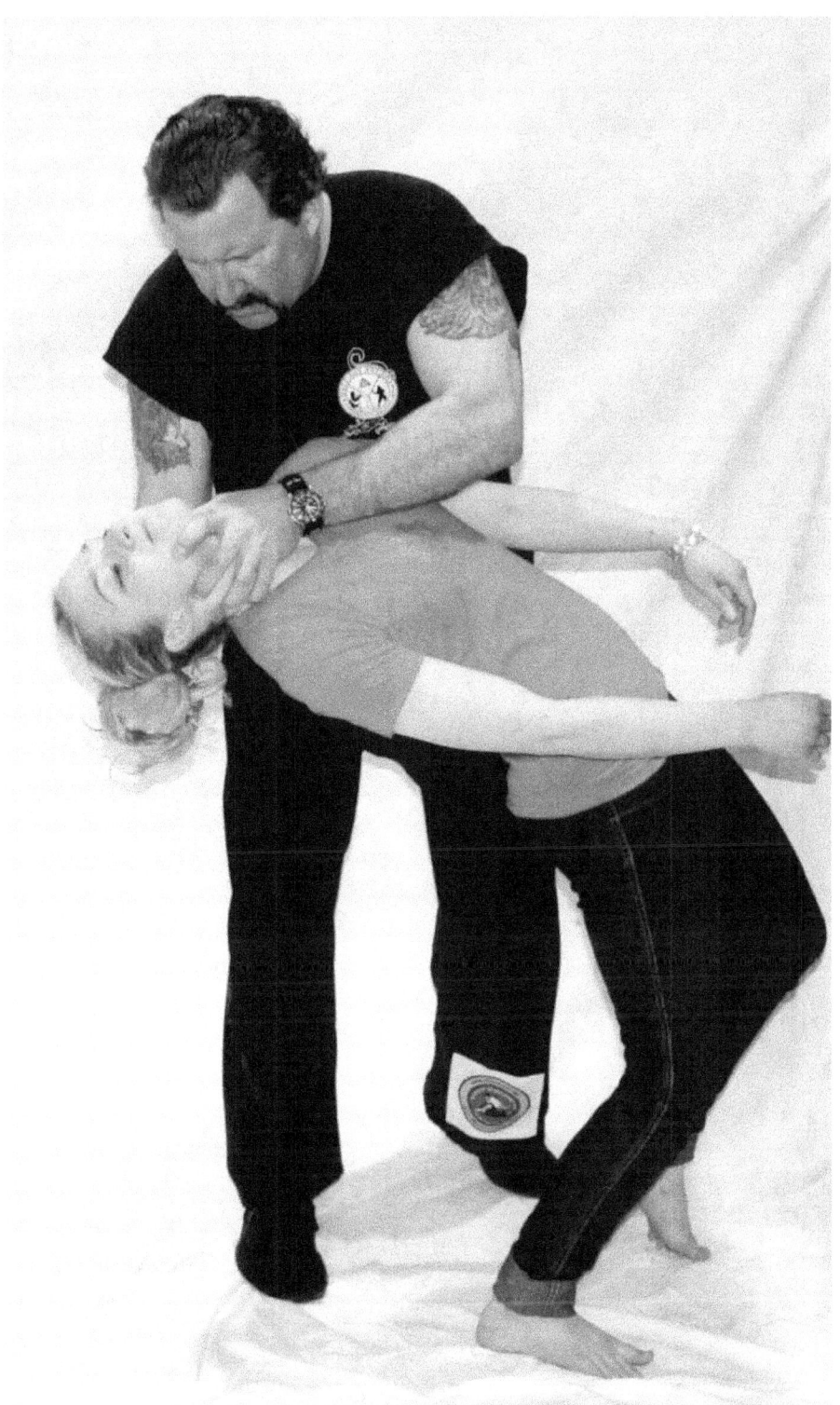

Don't be a victim!

Michael E. Andrus

www.ustaysafe.com

ISBN-10:149447414X
ISBN-13:978-1494474140

Printed in the U.S.A. 2014

First Edition

DEDICATION

I dedicate this book to past victims of violence. My commitment is to provide useful information that may save a life or prevent more victims. I wish everyone a Safe Day!

WARNING AND DISCLAIMER

The information and techniques in this book, when used properly, can provide you with the means to protect yourself and your loved ones from attackers. Be aware that the techniques contained herein could cause serious injury and even death. You are solely responsible for any and all use or misuse of these techniques. Please use the utmost caution when studying and practicing this material.

The author, demonstrators, photographers, producers, distributors and any others involved with this book are in no way responsible for the use or misuse of the material contained in this book.

The content of this book is solely the opinion of the author and is based on his many years of training in the area of practical self-defense. The author has researched all techniques demonstrated and presents the results to you in this book. The teaching in this book is for informational purposes only. Please train only with a qualified instructor.

Please consult a certified instructor before training in any martial art or engaging in any physical activity.

ACKNOWLEDGEMENTS

I would like to thank my parents, who have unconditionally supported my efforts, and my daughter Lauren, who has inspired me to make a difference. A special thanks to Annie for her enthusiasm, time and suggestions in helping me produce a quality product for my readers. Thank you to the many qualified and talented martial arts instructors who have shared their knowledge with me. I would like to thank my friend and fellow martial artist Jillian Santacroce, who appears in this book. Photography provided by Brian Smith at Brian's Pro Photos www.briansprophotos.com.

I am humbled and grateful to be able to share this knowledge with others that it may make a difference!

Michael E. Andrus

PREFACE

The world is changing every day. It's not the relaxed, safe place we once knew when we were children. There are many people among us who refuse to take responsibility for their actions. This attitude affects us all, especially our personal safety. These days, it is wise to understand your surroundings, have better awareness and be able to defend yourself if needed. Those who say, "It always happens to someone else, never me!" may regret those words if and when a tragedy strikes. Having the confidence in your ability to face our new culture is important for a happy and healthy life.

I have learned and developed effective techniques from many years of training in multiple styles of martial arts. For this book, I have selected what I feel to be the most practical self-defense techniques for women to use to defend themselves against an attacker who may be bigger and stronger.

I have put together a comprehensive program that teaches theory, dynamics and practical techniques for women's self-defense. My book, seminars, classes and workshops teach self-defense for individuals and their families. The training includes practical techniques designed to properly defend against attackers in a home invasion, car invasion and other scenarios related to real-world violence. My street-proven self-defense techniques also include awareness drills and tips to keep you out of trouble. Keen awareness, practical self-defense techniques and the confidence to protect yourself are necessary in today's world.

"Staying in the Moment!"

The concept of "staying in the moment" came about from my research of how women generally respond to danger events and why. Women are wired differently than men and are culturally taught to be open and engaging. This, however, does not work well in today's society. Women also have a flinch mechanism and usually close their eyes and turn away from danger or perceived danger. This reaction can cause a big problem, as you can guess! Turning away from something coming toward you can be very dangerous. You can't see what is happening, and you won't be able to respond properly to the situation.

By understanding the reactions, I was able to design my program to educate women and help them change the way they respond and react to external encounters. These encounters may be as simple as a conversation or they may be a more traumatic situation. The result is that by using the principles I teach, women are more confident and more aware of their surroundings. They can also respond properly and focus by "staying in the moment" to resolve the conflict.

The training involves some meditation, awareness drills, education, self-defense and "the element of surprise" techniques, as well as discussion about applying what you learn. Being able to apply what you learn is KEY!

The results have been amazing. We are finding that these principles and techniques can be used successfully in every area of our life. Women (anyone for that matter) can utilize these principles during medical exams, conversations with their boss or coworkers, when traveling and even at home with family and friends. The principles allow you to concentrate quickly and focus on what needs to done at that very moment. The result could be the difference between life and death!

Changing the way someone does things and the way they think isn't easy. You have to prove out your theory. I not only tell people, but I show them it works! When people see what works, they want to have the ability to be effective too.

What is interesting is that "staying in the moment" is not always about conflict resolution. By doing things with intent you can change the moment, the rest of your day, or the rest of your life! I hope those who read my book or take my workshops, seminars and classes take away a sense of "newfound ability". They always had what it takes; they just didn't know where to find it and how to put it all together. These principles help you focus, do things with intent and get the results you desire.

Wishing everyone a Safe Day!

Sincerely,

"Mr. Mike" "Taz" Andrus

Founder/Master Instructor

Safe Day Studio

ABOUT THE AUTHOR

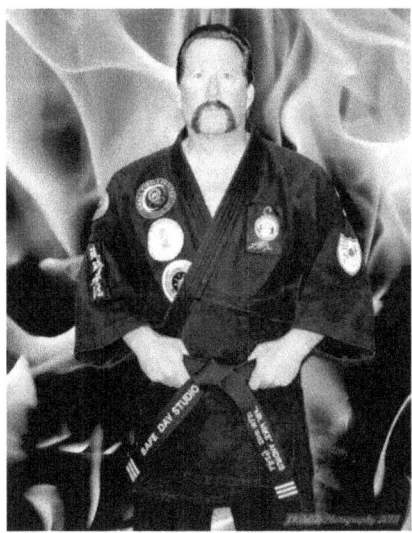

"Mr. Mike" "Taz" Andrus
Sho-Dai Soke
Founder/Master Instructor
Safe Day Studio

Mr. Mike's training and teaching experience with martial arts and self-defense goes back many years. He is responsible for the creation of all of the programs at Safe Day Studio. These programs include Hon Hab Do, Children's Karate, Mixed Martial Arts (MMA), traditional martial arts, practical self-defense and Brazilian Jiu-Jitsu. He also created and teaches "Teen Safety Techniques", "Women's Self-Defense" and "Rollin' with Safe Day", a wheelchair self-defense program for those who are challenged with Spina Bifida. He has achieved LFI (Lethal Force Institute) Level 1, taught privately. He has been an instructor for the World Karate Elite fighting system. He is the Master of Ceremonies and Ring Announcer for Friday Night Muay Thai fights at the Taj Mahal Casino and Muay Thai Friday Night Fights: The Strikers Cup.

Mr. Mike has taught countless seminars at events including World Karate Union Hall of Fame weekend, Legends of Martial Arts, Action Martial Arts Magazine Hall of Fame, Kung Fu & Karate Expo, Tenant High School for "College Living" and "Out On My Own" curriculum, Indian Creek's private clients, Bucks County and Montessori Academy. He was selected as Security Advisor for Kaplan Career Institute for public safety.

In addition to training and teaching, Mr. Mike has extensive experience in personal security. He has provided protection to executives and celebrities. Mr. Mike is a director of security for a high-end supper and night club, and security advisor/trainer for the top night club in the Bahamas. He is also Director of Security for many events annually, such as the Washington Crossing Brewfest, Southampton Days, Newtown Beerfest, Brews & Bites at Pennsbury Manor, Warminster Days, and the Bucks County Fireman's parade and festival. He has done armed undercover security for special events including high-end jewelry trunk shows. He has also taught law enforcement and military tactical training and is a lethal weapons agent (Act 235) in Pennsylvania and a cybersecurity advisor for the Federal Agents PBA.

Because of his training and experience, Mr. Mike has been asked to speak to a variety of audiences, including the Bucks County Meta-physical Society, the Christian's Women's Club, the North Penn Chamber of Commerce, Montgomery County Community College, Girl Scouts of America, for whom he also created the self-defense merit badge program in Bucks County, Women's networking groups and Kappa Sigma Fraternity at Temple University. He was also the primary subject matter expert for, "The Benefits of Martial Arts for Women" an article published in Diet and Nutrition Magazine. He is the self-defense expert at the Philly Fit retreats in Avalon, NJ and was the Director of the 1st Annual BJJ Tournament at the 2010 WKUHOF Weekend.

Mr. Mike currently holds public and private women's self-defense seminars, and in addition to this book, he is filming a 4-part DVD involving personal responsibility and intent, titled "Staying in the Moment!"

AWARDS

2013 International Circle of Masters Hall of Fame inductee and "Grand Master Instructor of the Year"

2013 Chinese Kung Fu & Karate Expo – Martial Arts Master Lifetime Achievement Award

2013 Legends of Martial Arts Hall of Fame inductee and "Master of the Year for Reality-Based Self-Defense"

2012 I.A.M.A. (International Association of Martial Arts) Hall of Fame inductee

2012 World Karate Hall of Fame "Outstanding Contribution to Women's Self-Defense Program"

2010, 2011, 2012, 2013 Action Martial Arts Magazine Hall of Honors Inductee "Good

Will Ambassador for Exemplary Contributions to the Martial Arts"

2010, 2011 World Karate Union Hall of Fame "Most Distinguished Board Member of the Year"

2010 Action Martial Arts Magazine Hall of Honors inductee "Outstanding Contributions to the Martial Arts"

2010 Hall of Recognition – GNPRBFI (Global Network of Professional Reality-Based Fighting Instructors) "Instructor of the Year" for Women's Self Defense

2009 GNPRBFI (Global Network of Professional Reality-Based Fighting Instructors) - Board Member/Certified Instructor/Advisor

2009 World Karate Hall of Fame Board of Director

2008 World Karate Union Hall of Fame inductee

2008 World Karate Union Hall of Fame "Instructor of the Year" for Mixed Martial Arts & Hon Hab Do

2007 Safe Day Studio voted, "Best School of 2007" by AWMA (Asian World of Martial Arts)

You can contact the author at:

Safe Day Studio

Phone: 215-370-1650
Email: info@ustaysafe.com
www.info@ustaysafe.com

Michael E. Andrus

CONTENTS

Michael E. Andrus

CHAPTER 1

STAY IN THE MOMENT: FACE-TO-FACE CONFRONTATION

Quick, effective techniques to protect against an attack from the front

Scenario: You have finished a successful day of shopping at the mall and are thrilled with your new purchases. As you walk through the parking lot, you realize that you're running late for your dinner plans. You are looking through your purse for your cell phone to text a quick apology to your friend when you notice a man walking toward you. You have an uneasy feeling as he continues to approach you. At the last moment, he lunges toward you. What do you do?

Technique #1: "The Wedge"

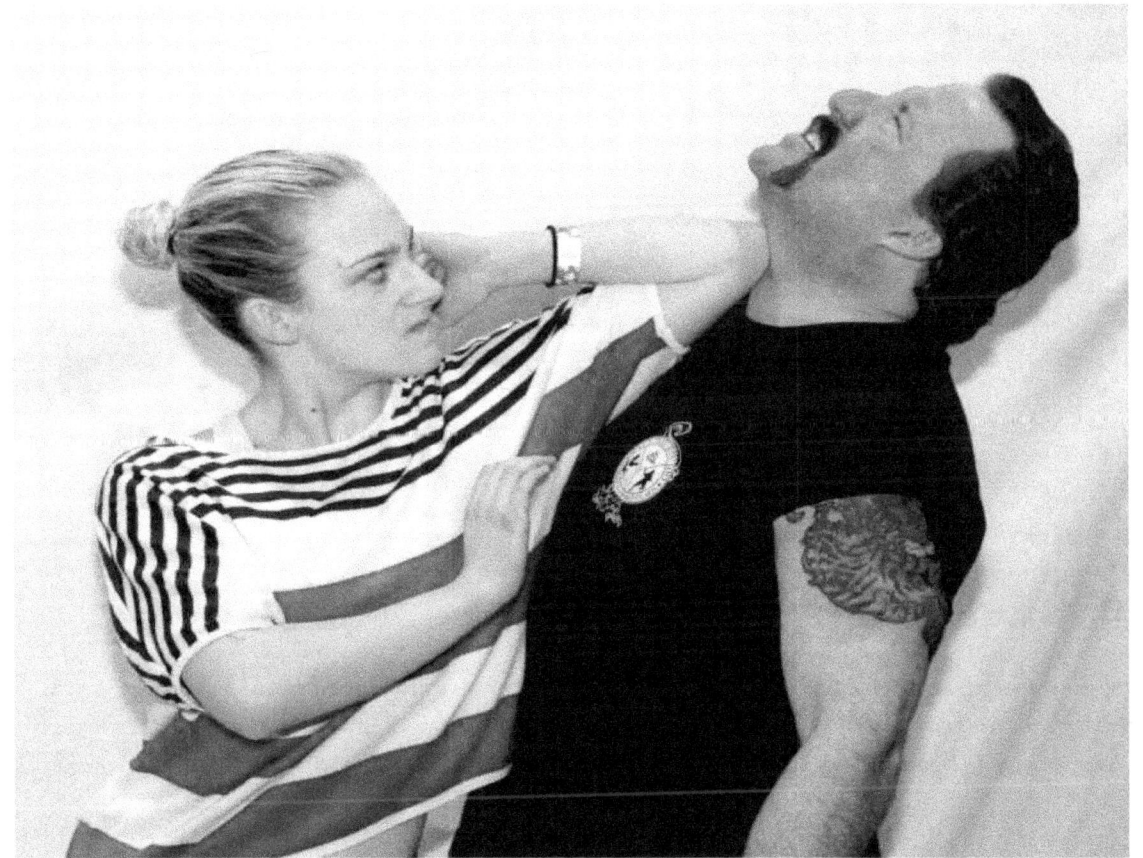

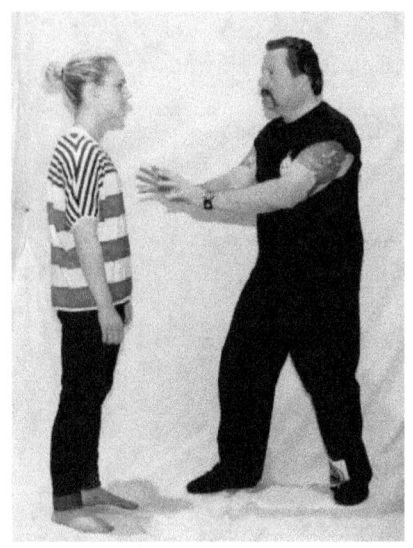

Attacker attempts to grab your arms or neck with one or both hands

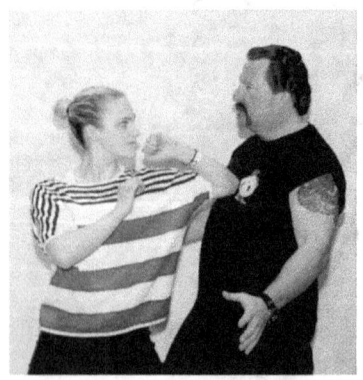 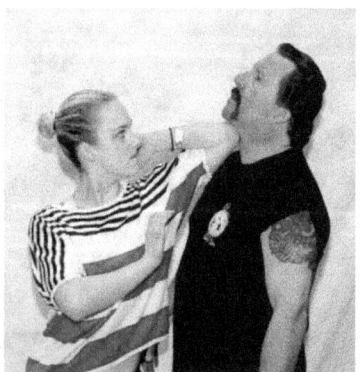 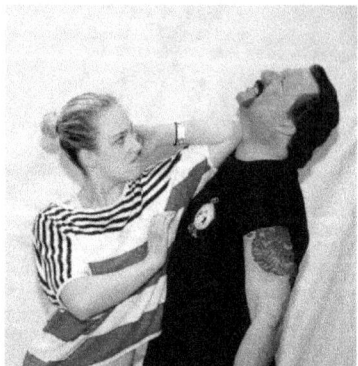

Step forward driving your elbow into attacker's chest. The strike should be as hard as you can as you step forward, using the bony part of your elbow. The strike is straight into the sternum/solar plexus (center of chest). Snap elbow up sharply into throat then under chin (may cut off part of the attacker's tongue).

You have several options after the wedge strike to the sternum and throat:

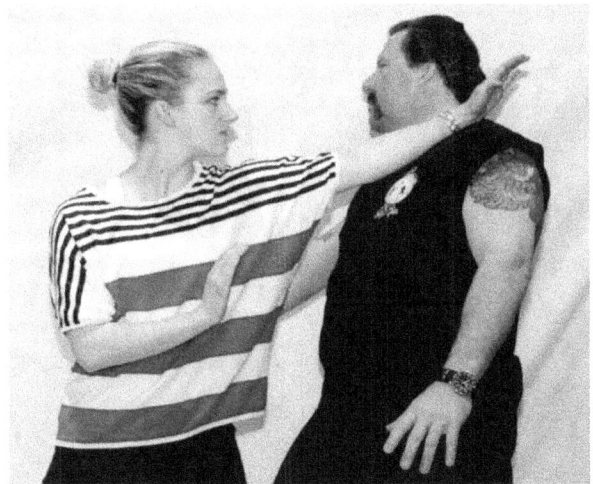

a) Right side of neck/head strike, which keeps the attacker out of your centerline.

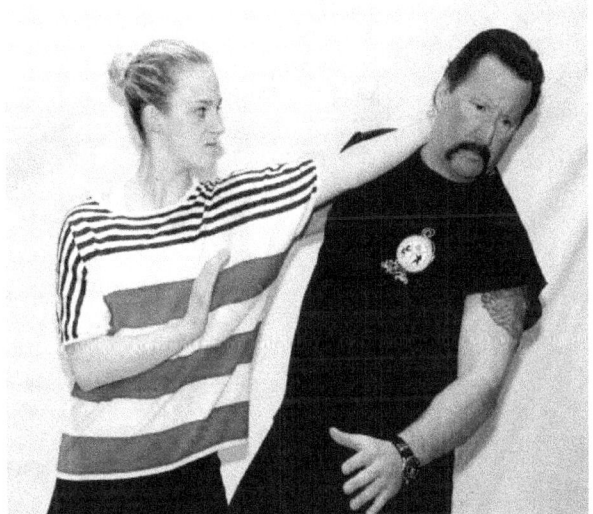

b) Left side of neck/head strike, which opens attacker up to additional strikes to head, neck, body and groin.

How to deliver an effective kick to the groin

You may think that a knee to the groin is the safest and most effective kick. You'd be wrong! You may be successful using your knee at a very close range.

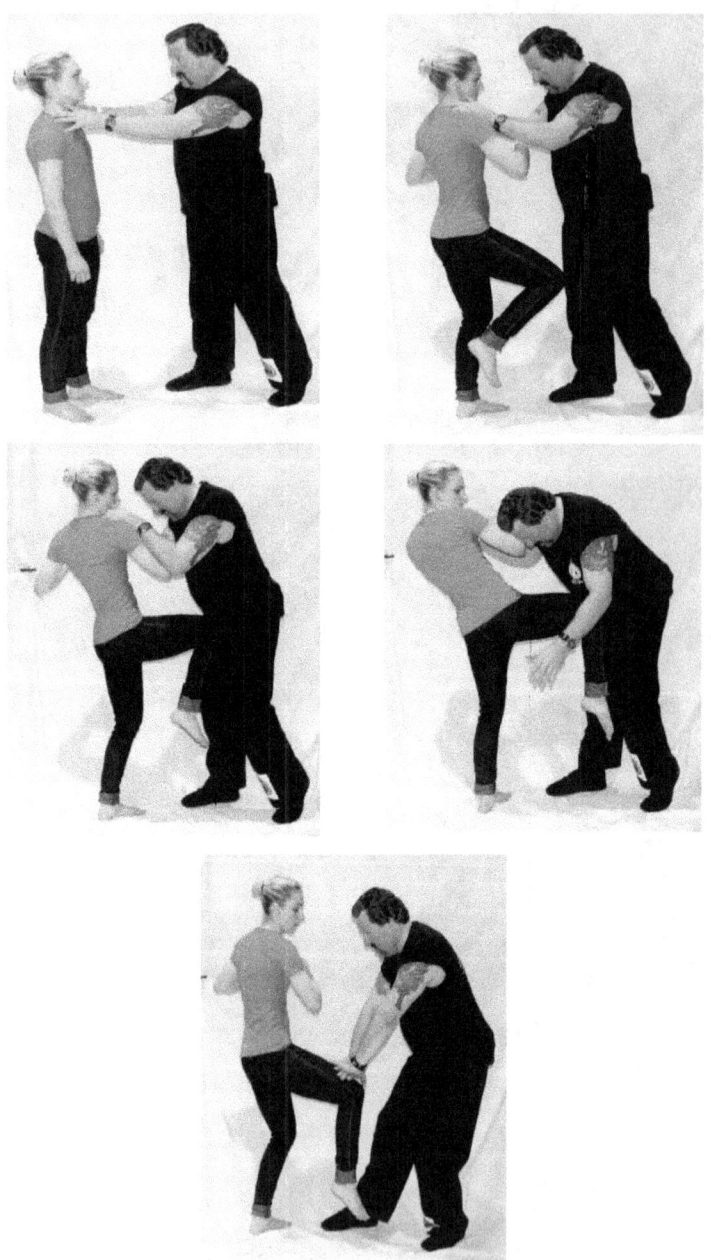

However, the attacker may be able to grab your leg or use his hands to block your knee thrust.

Straight-leg kick to the groin - An effective option that works!

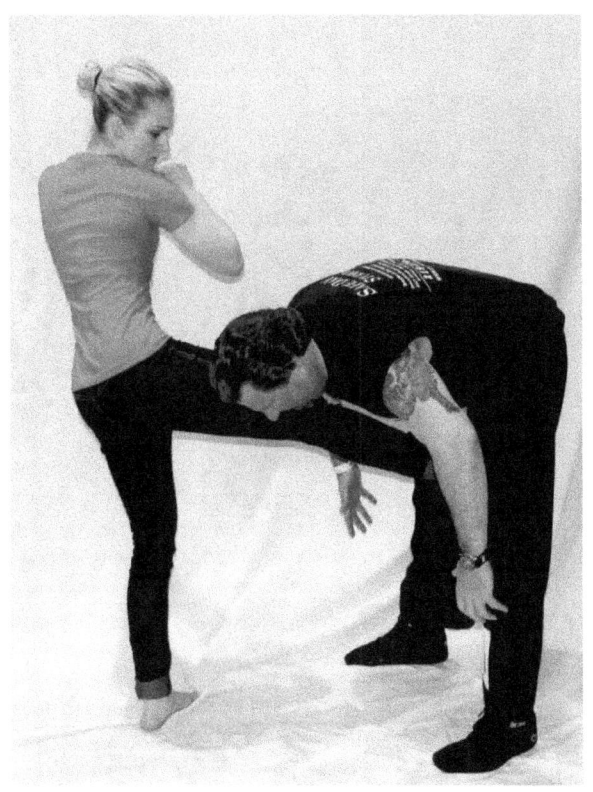

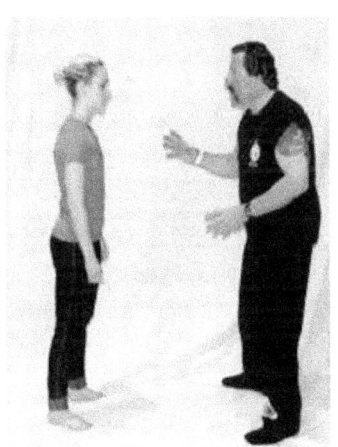 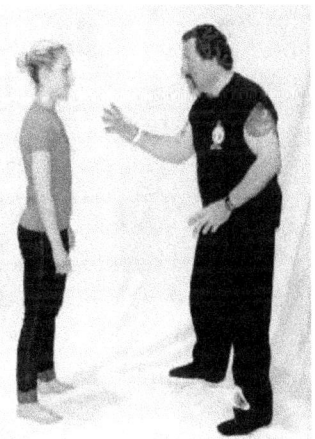 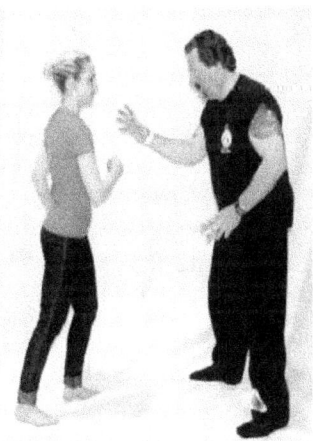

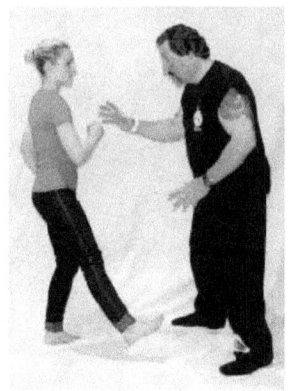 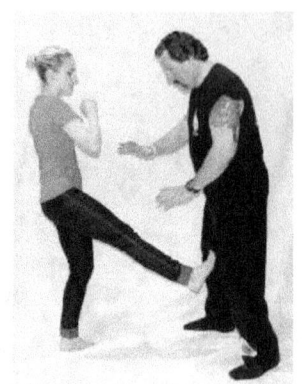

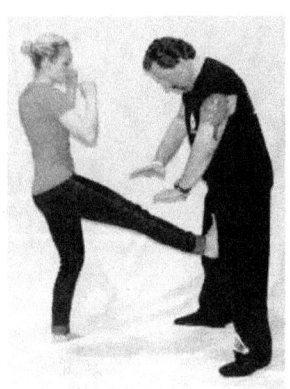 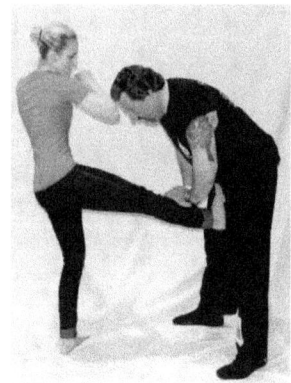 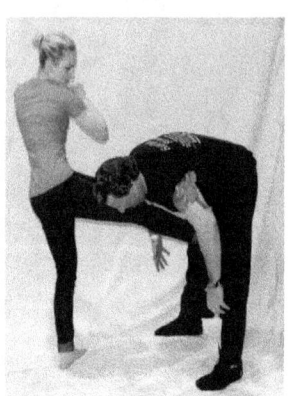

Keeping your leg straight, continue to kick up under the attacker's hands and drive your foot up into the attacker's groin. You are striking the underside of the attacker's groin area, which is extremely painful and may disable the attacker. A pointed, hard shoe is ideal for this kick. It is very difficult for an attacker to block this straight-leg kick. Even if his arms are stretched out and down, this technique hits its target.

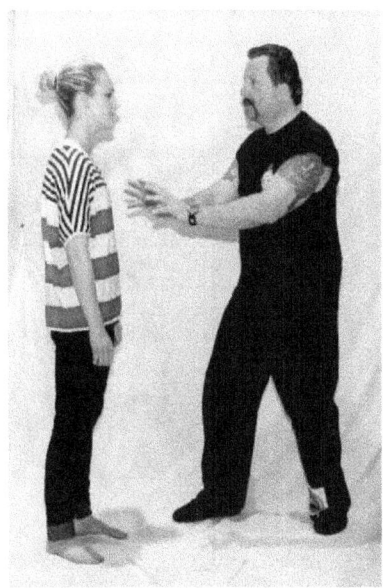

Attacker attempts to grab your chest or neck with one or both hands

Technique #2: The Chin

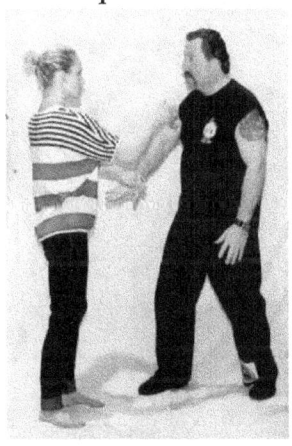 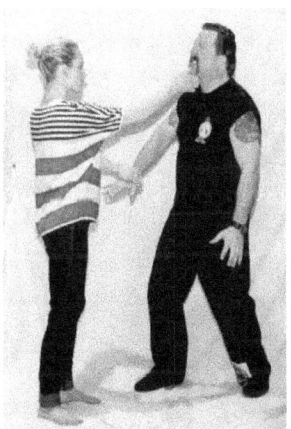 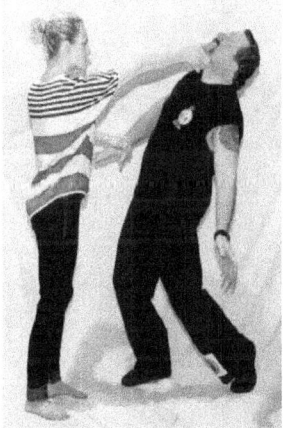

Take your thumb nail and drive it straight into the attacker's chin below the lip. Push hard in and down. Don't forget to use your nail!

Technique #3: The Cheek

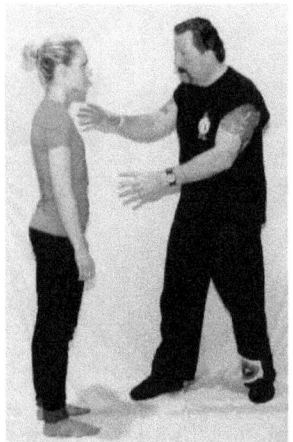 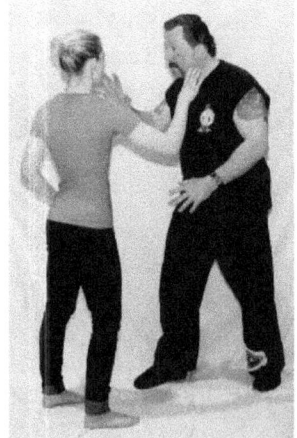 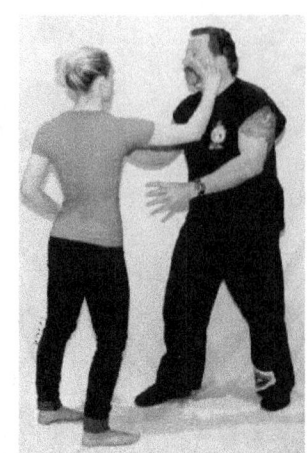

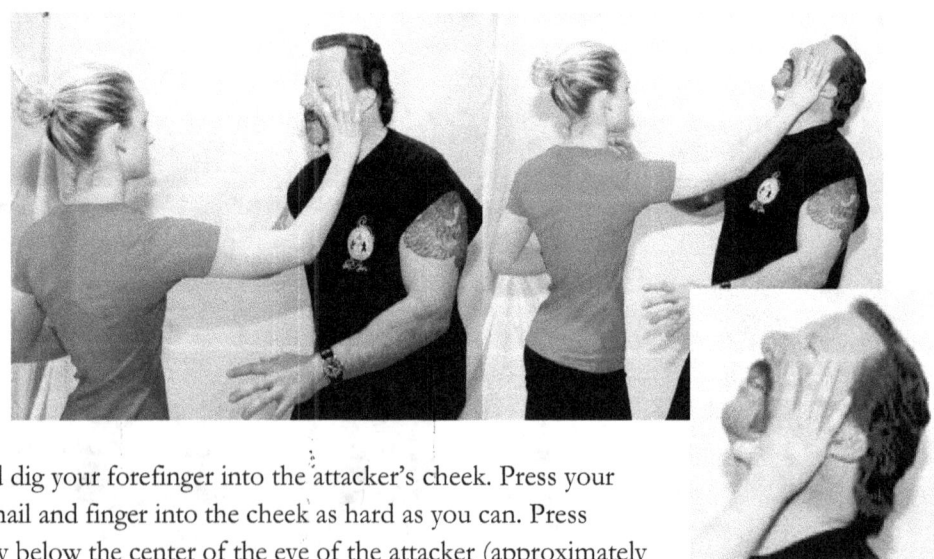

Reach
up and dig your forefinger into the attacker's cheek. Press your
fingernail and finger into the cheek as hard as you can. Press
directly below the center of the eye of the attacker (approximately
2 inches below the eye). Dig and push the attacker's face back away
from you and down towards the ground.

Note: This technique opens up the attacker's throat which becomes a
target for you to punch. Punch the attacker's throat with a closed fist.
You can also use an open hand thrust using your fingers to jab the
attacker's throat. You can also kick the attacker in the groin.

Technique #4: The Ear

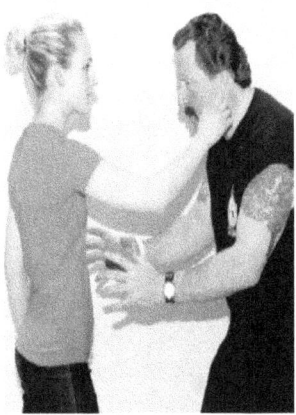 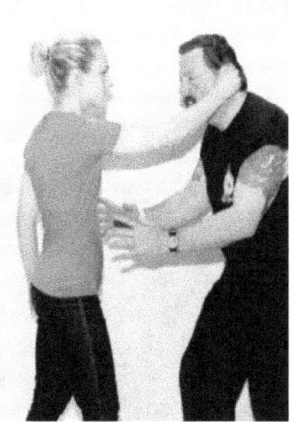 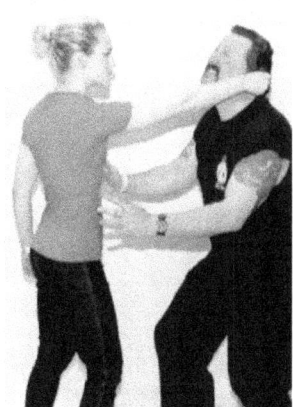

As the attacker attempts to grab you, reach up and grab the attacker's ear. Grab the attacker's entire ear with your hand. Squeeze your hand and dig your nails into to attacker's ear while doing this technique. As you grab and squeeze the attacker's ear, bend the ear away from you and down.

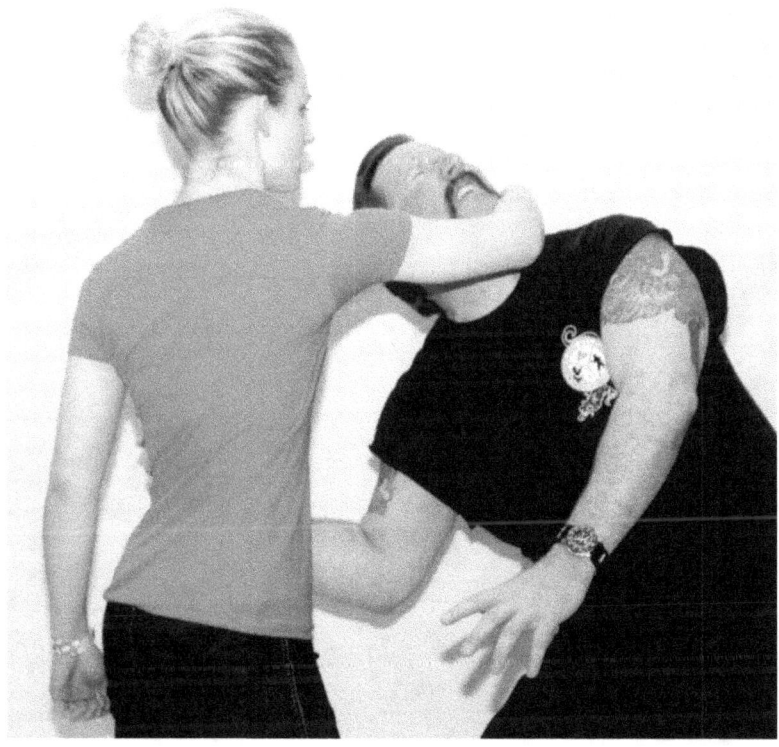

After you bend the ear away from you and push down, turn the attacker's head to the side. (Snap the attacker's head to the left using your right hand or snap the attacker's head to the right if you're using your left hand.)

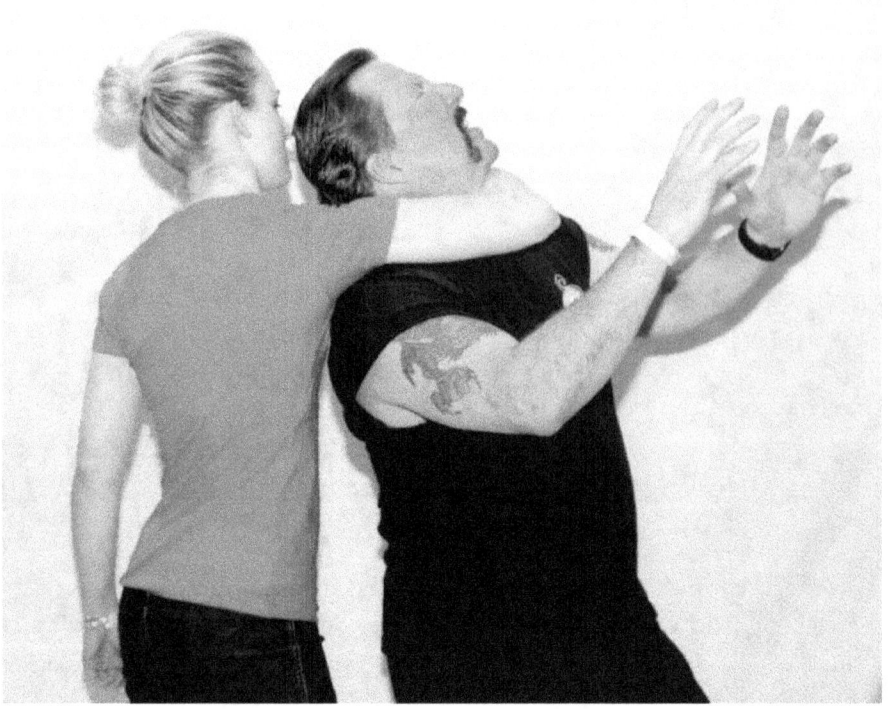

You can now escape or do any or all of the following:

    a) Choke the attacker.

    b) Rake the attacker's eyes and face with your hand and nails.

    c) Kick or knee the attacker in the legs, kidneys or back.

    d) Punch the attacker in the back of the neck.

Technique #5: The Throat

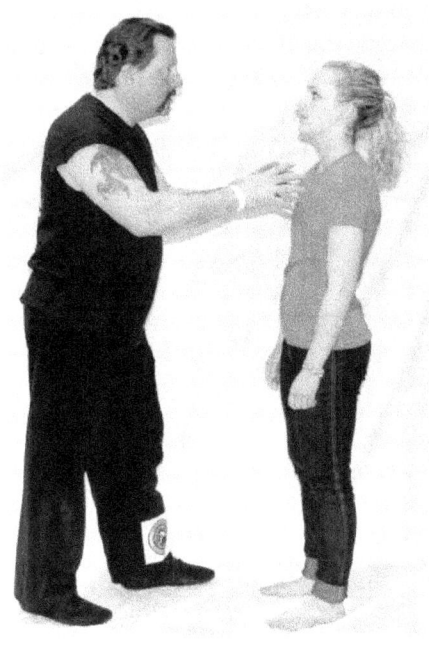

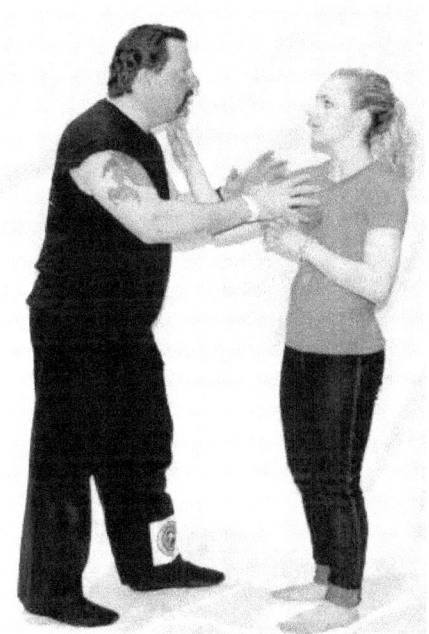 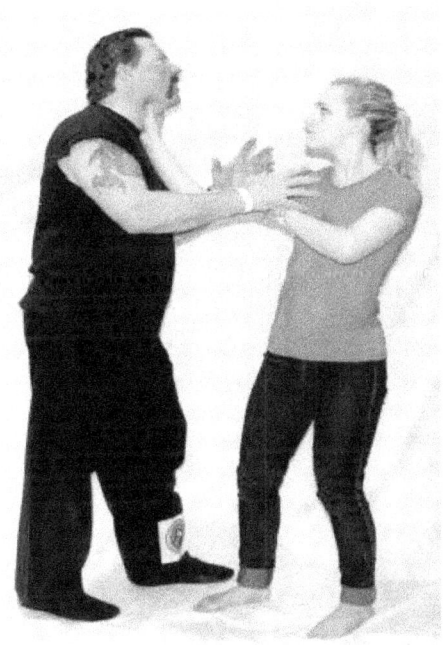

Reach up with both hands towards the attacker. Keep your hands inside the attacker's hands and grab his throat firmly. Dig your thumb into the attacker's throat behind the windpipe (Adam's apple) and turn your thumb inwards in an attempt to grab the windpipe. Place your hand and other four fingers flat against the neck. Squeeze has hard as you can!

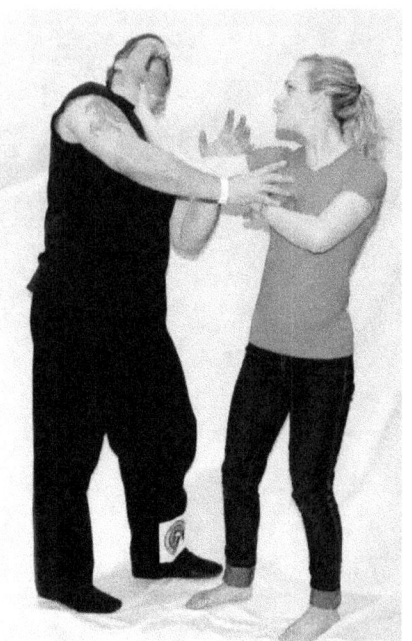 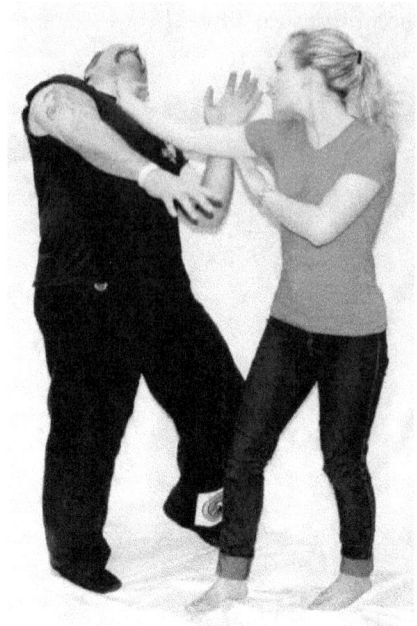

While applying the choke to the attacker, firmly push your hand away from you. This gives you room to escape.

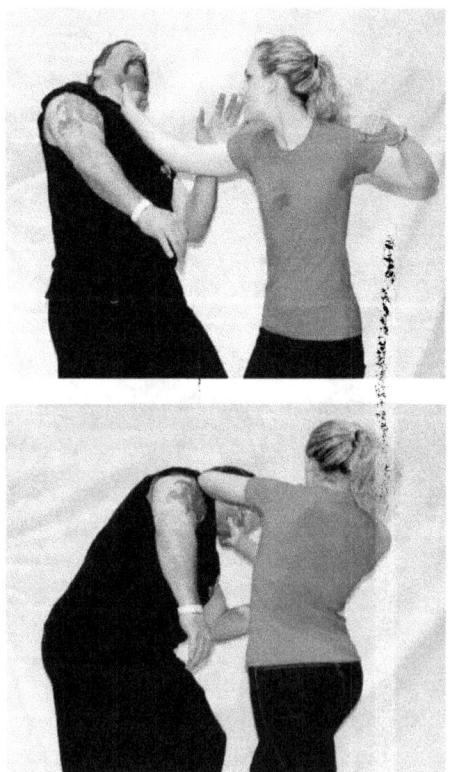 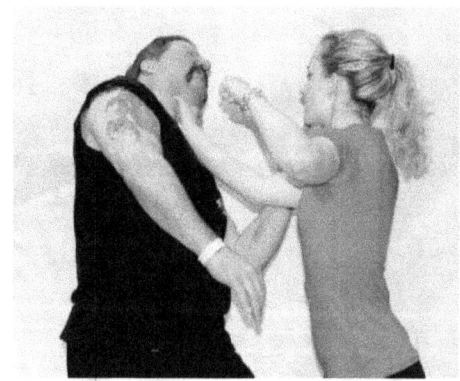

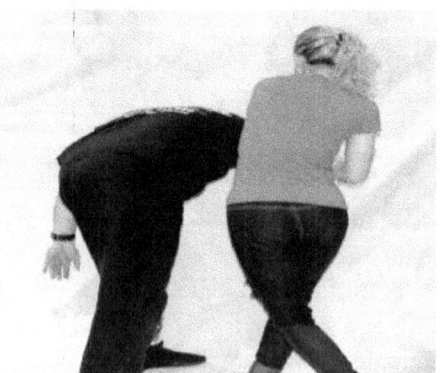

This technique may give you an opportunity to set up a direct punch to the throat or face of the attacker.

Technique #6: Multiple Strike Series 1 (Head Butt/Knee Strike/Front Kick)

Attacker attempts to grab you around the neck or chest.

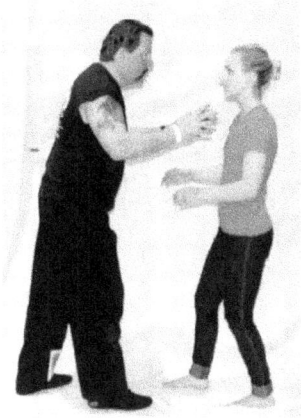 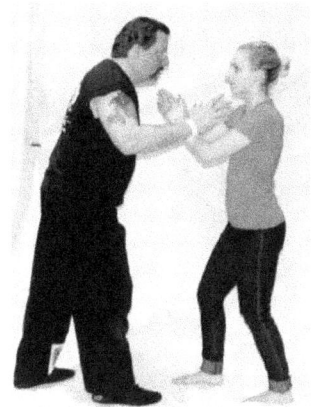 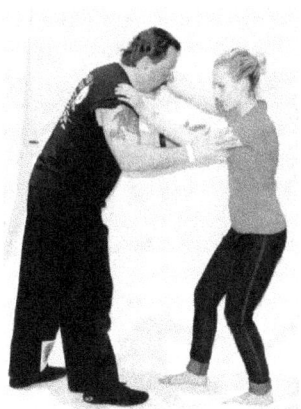

Bring your hands up inside the arms of the attacker. Reach up and get a firm grip on his shoulders, neck or back of head.

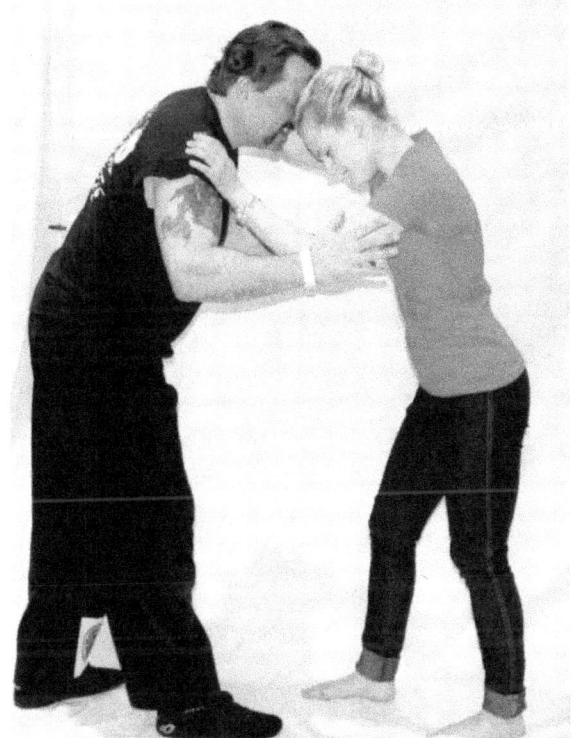

Head Butt - Tighten up your shoulders and neck. Then using your legs to push forward, drive your head into the attacker's face. You want to strike the attacker using the region of your head that is right above your hairline. Striking the nose region will get the best results. The attacker's eyes will water and this strike may leave them disoriented. Do this move as many times as you feel necessary.

Note: Do not use your nose or forehead to head butt the attacker—you will hurt yourself!

Knee Strike

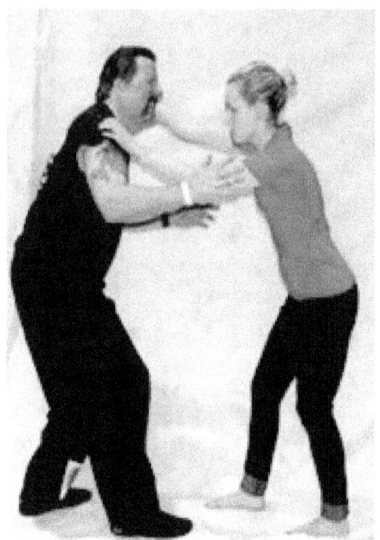 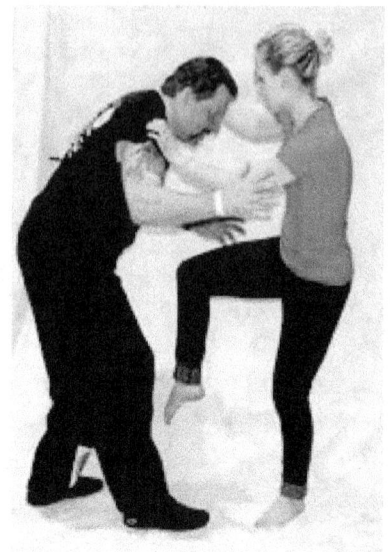

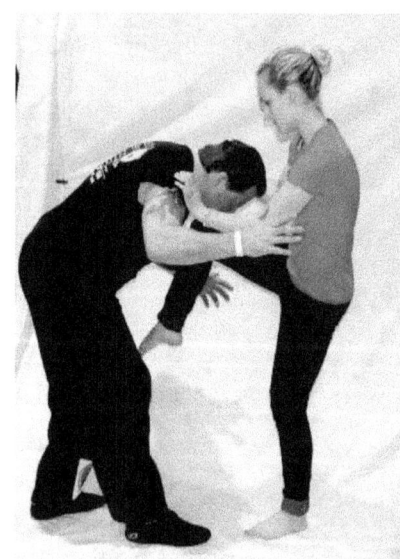

After you head butt the attacker, pull his head/shoulders/neck (whatever you can grab) down as hard as you can. Use your knee to strike him in the face again. Push your foot off the ground for extra power and momentum, and pull your knee up into the attacker's face as hard as you can.

Front Kick

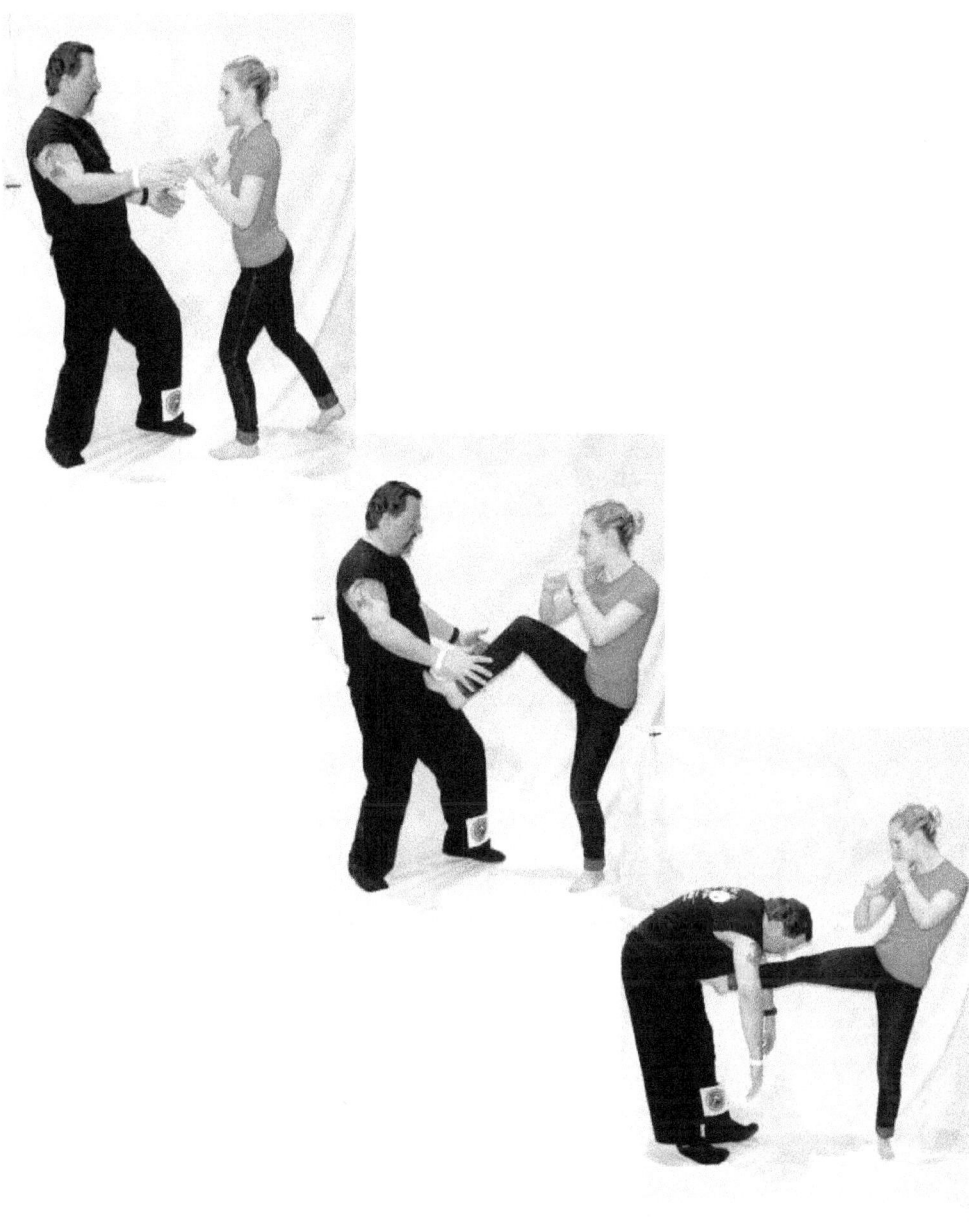

You can now kick the attacker in the groin, stomach or face. Use the ball of your foot when using a front kick. You may have the opportunity to use the tip of your shoe as well. Repeat this kick as many times as you feel necessary.

Technique #7: Multiple Strike Series 2 (Elbow Strike/Throat Strike/Knee Strike)

Attacker attempts to grab you around the waist or chest.

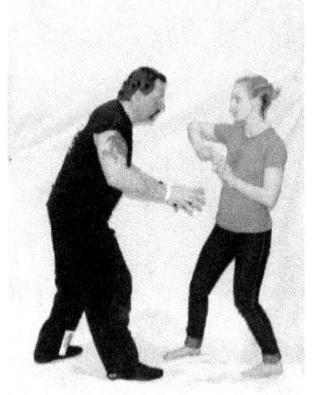 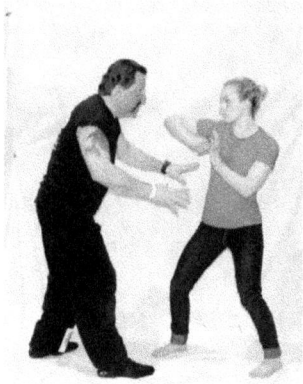 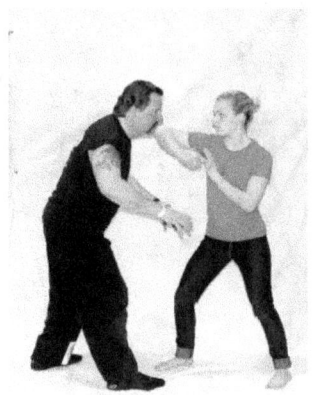

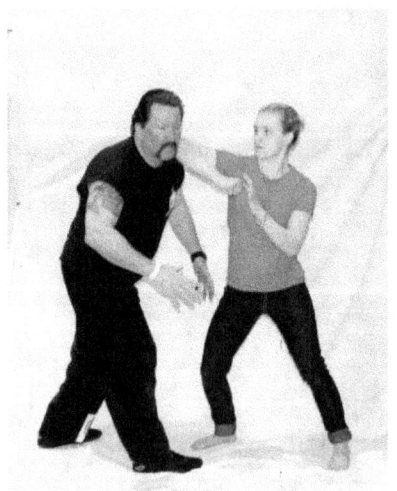 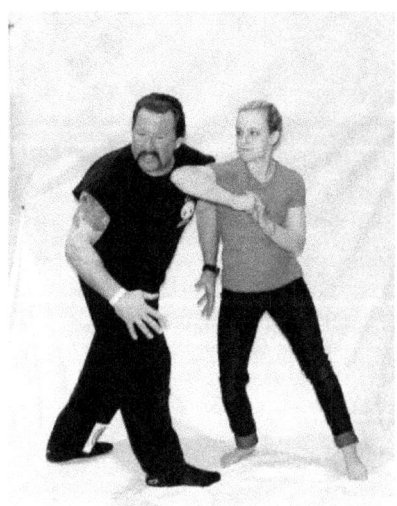

As the attacker reaches for you, step in with your right foot and drive your elbow into the attacker's jaw. There is a pressure point on the jaw bone that can knock out the attacker. This spot is located on the jawbone directly below the outer edge of the mouth.

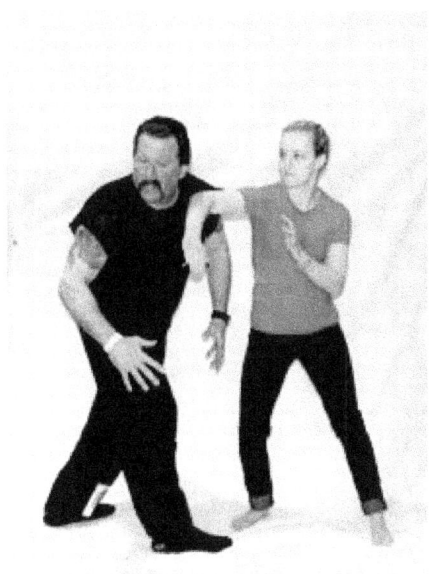 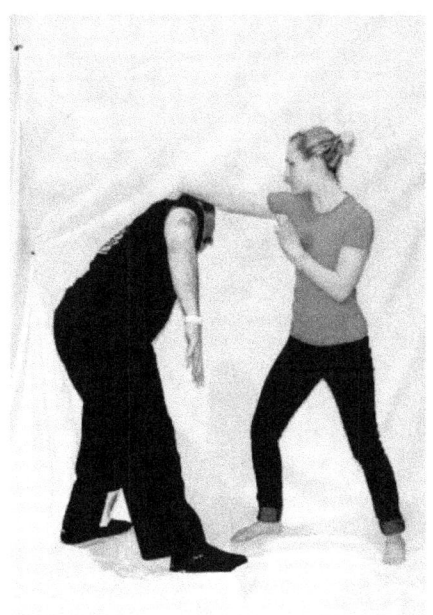

After your elbow strike, extend your arm and chop your hand back towards the attacker's throat. Strike the attacker's throat as hard as you can.

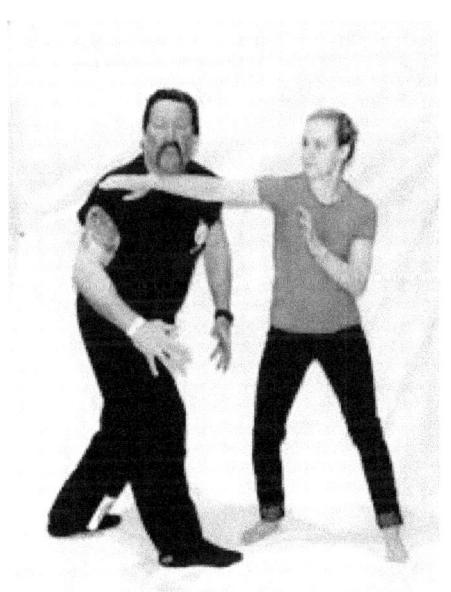 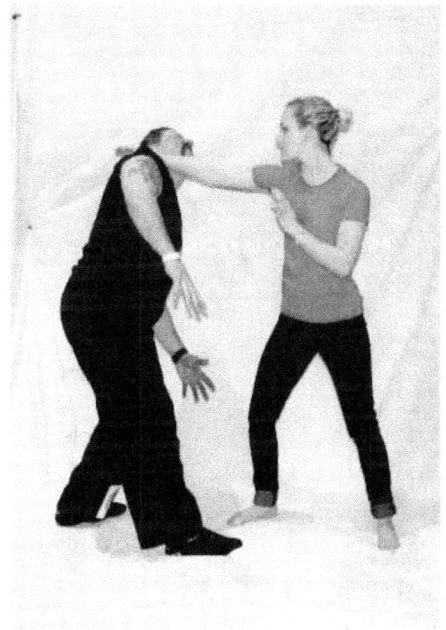

As you are following through with the throat strike, push the attacker's head down towards your knee.

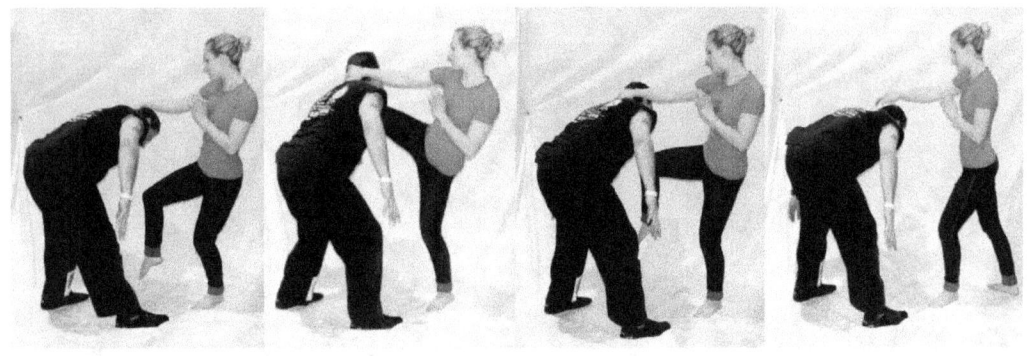

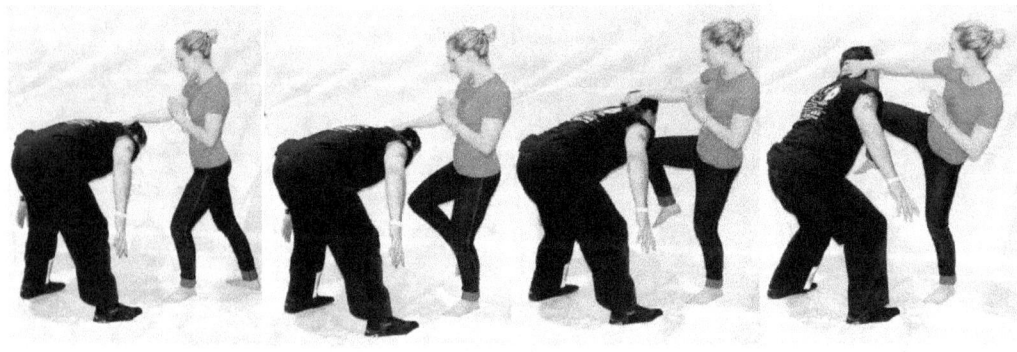

As you push the attacker's head down, drive your knee up into the attacker's nose. Repeat this as many times as you feel necessary. Continue to guide the attacker's head while doing this technique.

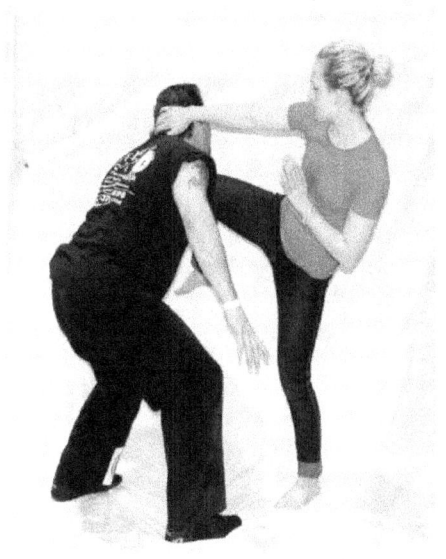 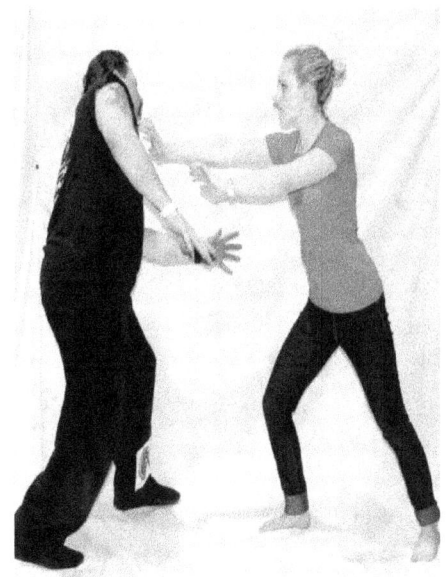

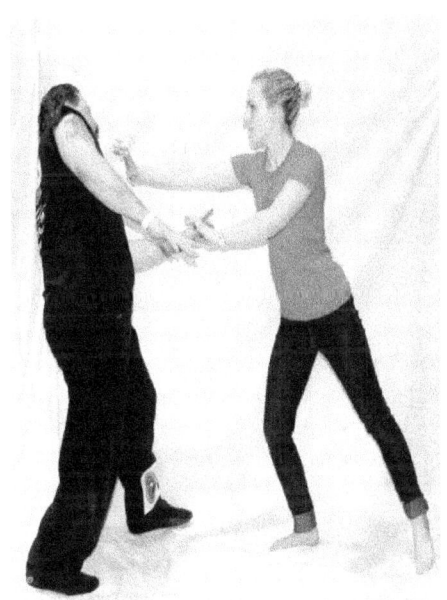 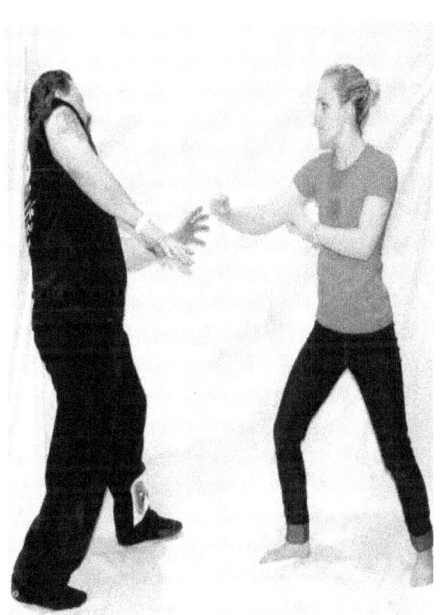

You can now push the attacker away from you and get into a fighting position.

Note: You can escape or continue different techniques. You are in a position to drive a strong front kick to the attacker's groin.

Technique #8: Multiple Strike Series 3 (Hammer Strike/Knee Strike/Elbow Strike/Front Kick)

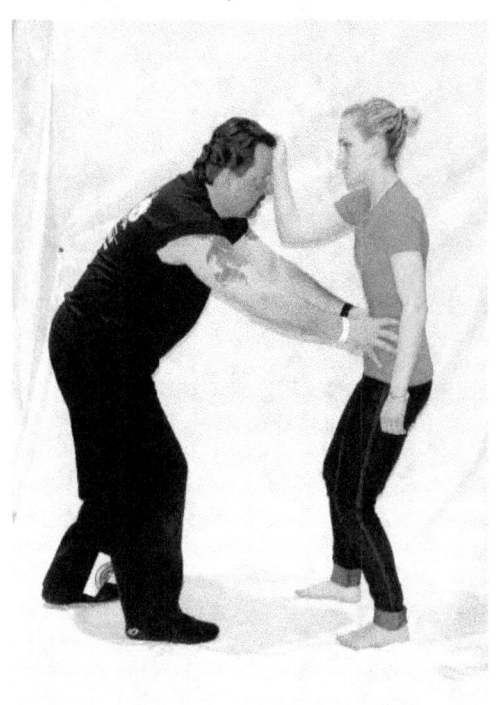

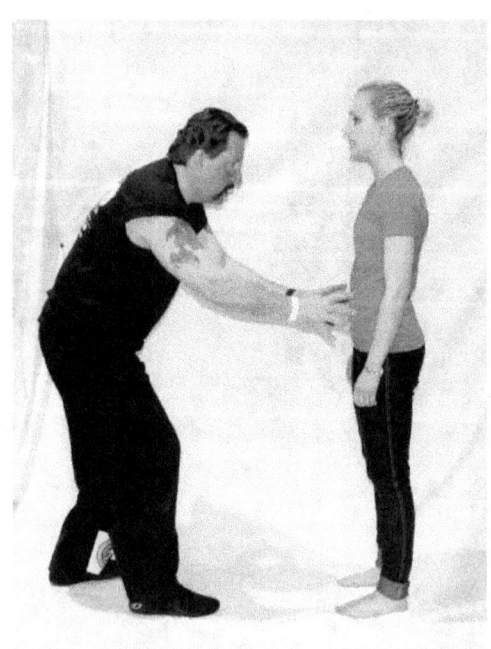

Attacker attempts to grab you around the waist.

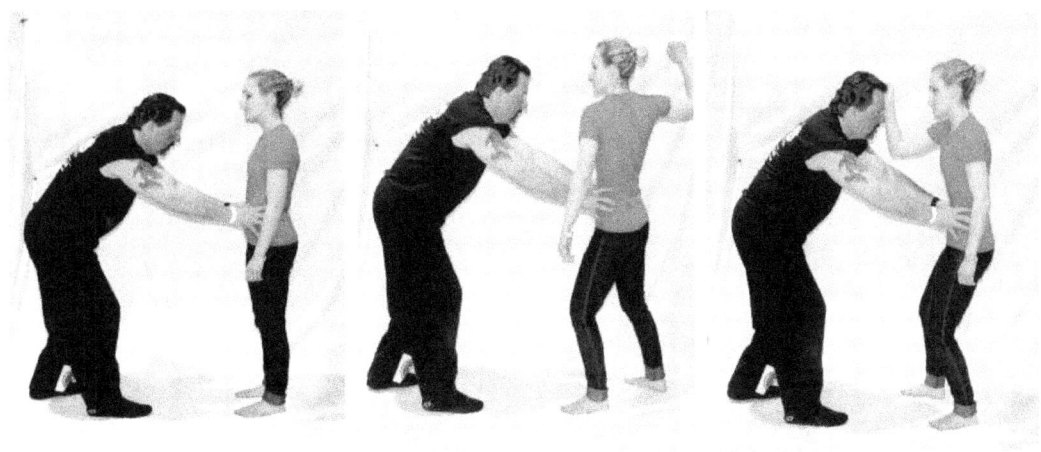

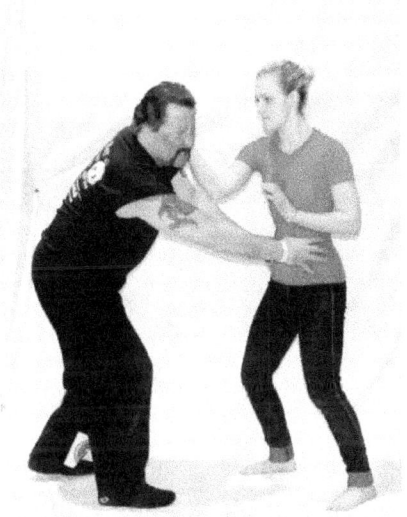
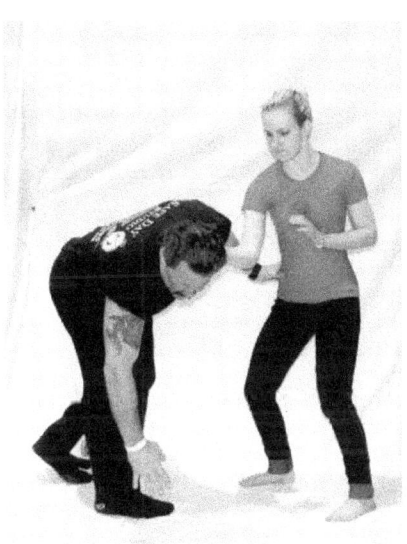

As the attacker reaches for your waist or chest step back and make a fist. Step forward and slam your fist into the attacker's head (on or behind his ear) as hard as you can. You must follow through with the fist strike.

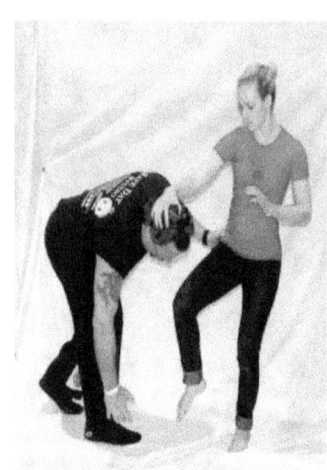

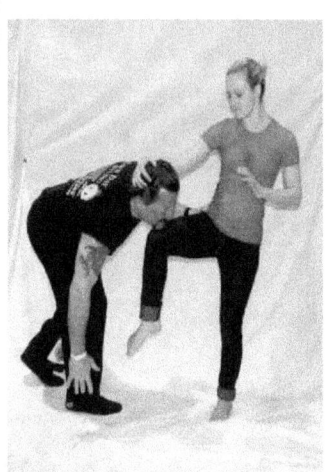

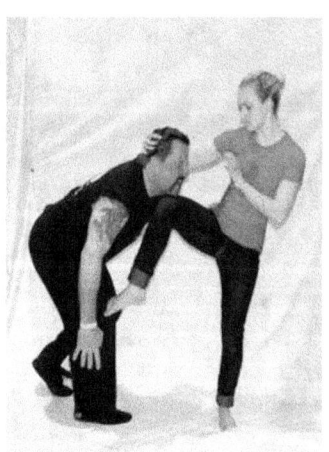

After you finish the hammer strike, grab the back of the attacker's head and push it down. As you push the attacker's head down, drive your knee up into the attacker's face. (The nose region will give you the most effective results).

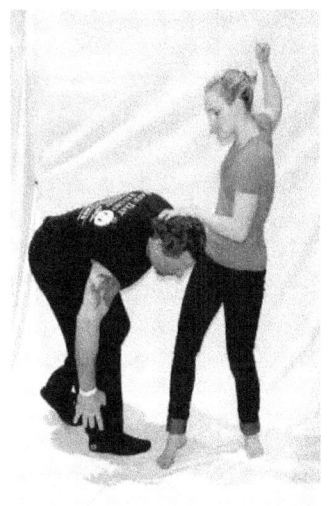 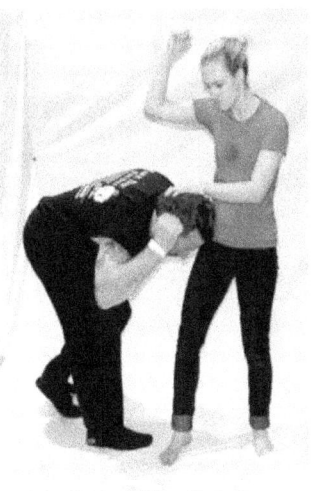 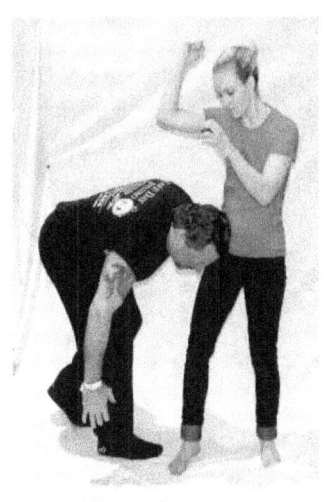

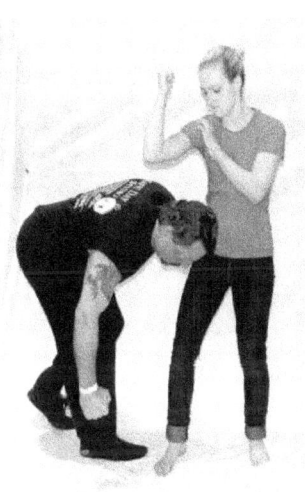 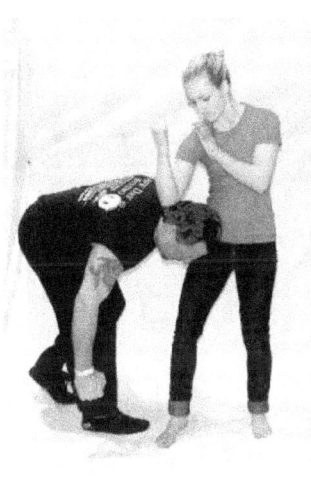 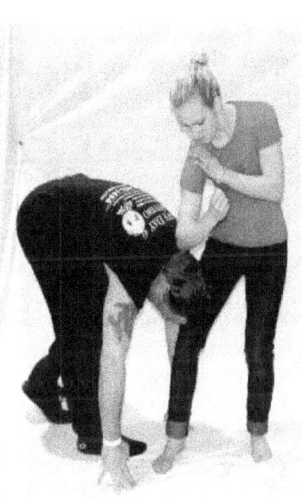

As you finish driving your knee up into the attacker's face, raise your hand and drive your elbow down into the back of the attacker's neck. You want your elbow to strike the attacker's neck directly behind his throat. This region is the C-5 vertebrae. Make sure this elbow strike is done as hard as you can.

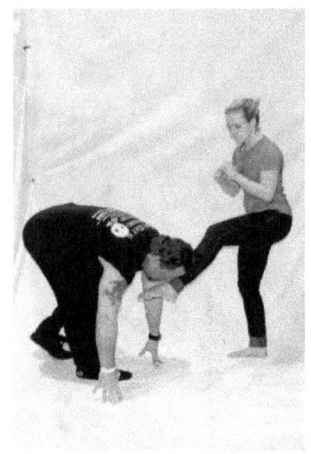

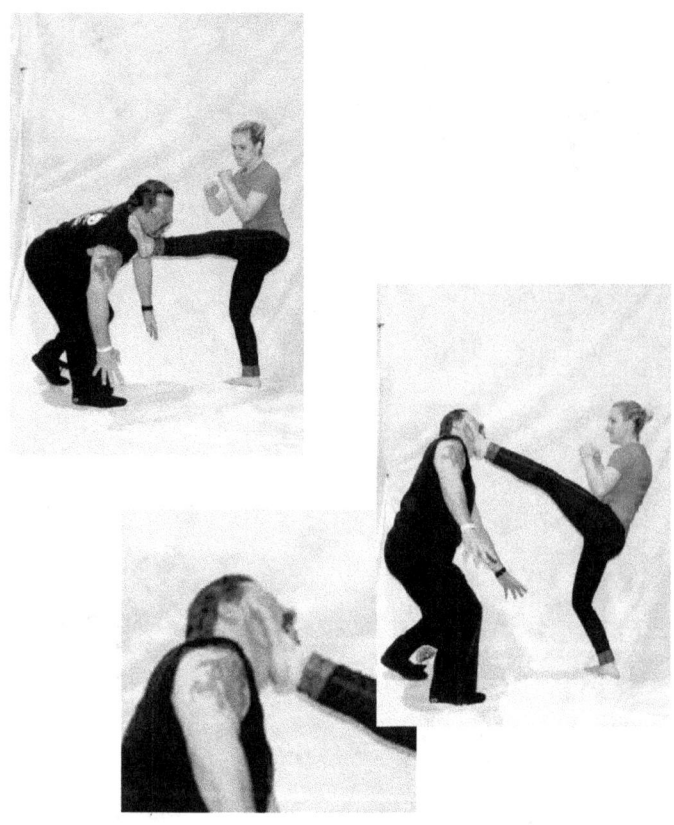

As you finish your elbow strike, the attacker's head will be down and forward, which gives you the opportunity to kick the attacker in the face. Using a modified front kick, kick as hard as you can. You will kick the attacker's face using the top of your foot and/or lower shin. Kicking the nose region will give you the most effective results.

CHAPTER ONE TIPS:

- Stay in the moment. If you get in trouble, stay calm, breathe and focus on staying safe.

- Look confident and alert. Pay attention to your surroundings and walk with purpose. Don't text or be otherwise distracted while walking.

- Use the element of surprise on your attacker to escape or protect yourself. For example, acting submissive may lead the attacker to let his guard down, which may give you the opportunity to execute a more effective counter-attack.

- Don't make direct eye contact with your attacker, which will actually cause you to freeze up. Instead, look at his nose, which will allow you to observe details for identification without distracting you. Try to get a description including facial shape, color of hair/eyes, clothing, scars/tattoos, direction they headed.

- Choose your parking space carefully. It is worth a longer walk to park in a well-lit area and to avoid parking in deserted alleys. Do not park next to vans with sliding doors.

- If an attacker asks for your wallet or handbag, throw it as fast and far away from you in one direction as possible while running in the other.

- Try to escape. If you can't, you must fight. If you fight, you do so to stay alive and survive!

CHAPTER 2

BE PREPARED: THE UNSEEN ATTACKER

Quick, effective techniques to protect against an attack from the rear

Scenario: You are enjoying a happy hour drink when a guy at the bar strikes up a conversation with you. At first, you try to discourage him without being rude. Ultimately, he refuses to take the hint, and even begins to get hostile with you for rejecting his advances. Rather than engage with him further, you pay your tab and leave the bar, assuring your friends you'll call them when you get home. You're walking to your car when he comes up behind you. What do you do?

Attacker attempts to grab you from behind in a bear hug.

Technique #9: "Going on Vacation"

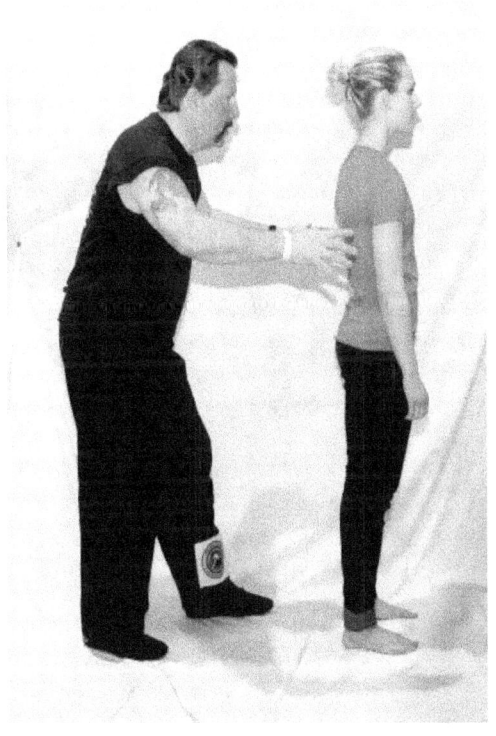 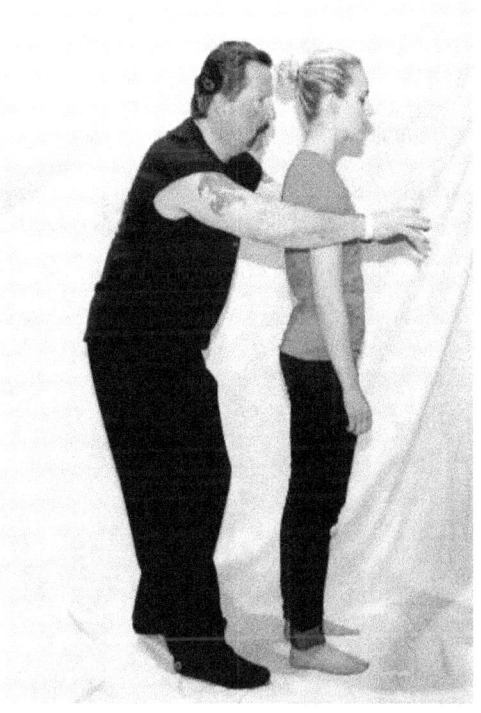

The attacker approaches you from the rear trying to wrap his arms around you, hug and control you.

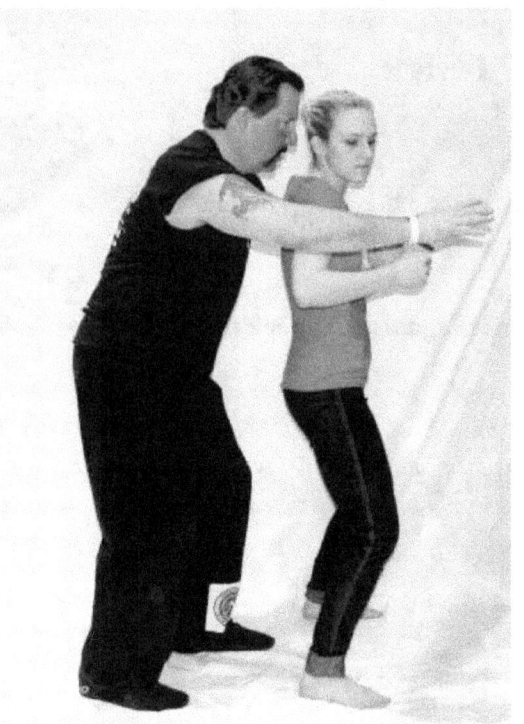

Step to the left side slightly with your left foot so you have a good solid stance. Extend your arm forward like you're reaching for a door knob.

Drive your elbow straight back hard into the attacker's solar plexus (center of the chest) as if you're pulling open a stuck door open.

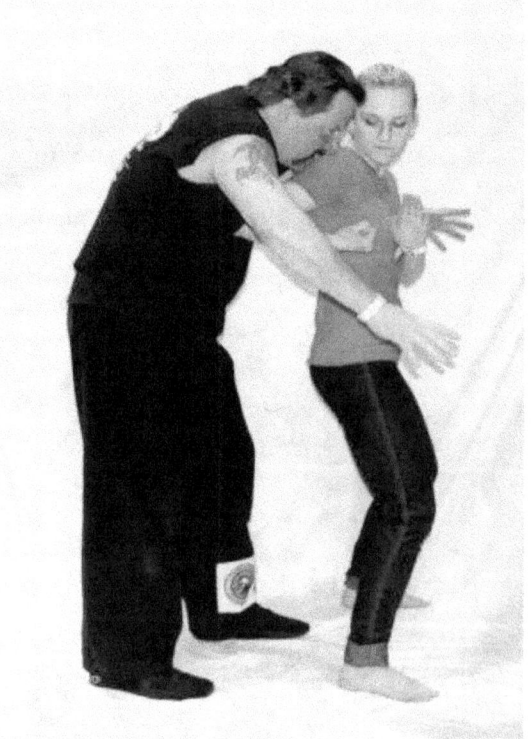

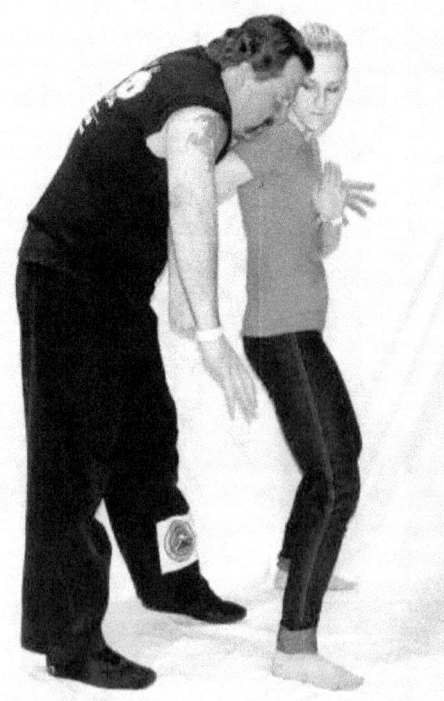

While keeping your elbow in the attacker's chest region, punch down with a closed fist to the attacker's groin, as if you're reaching down to pick up your luggage.

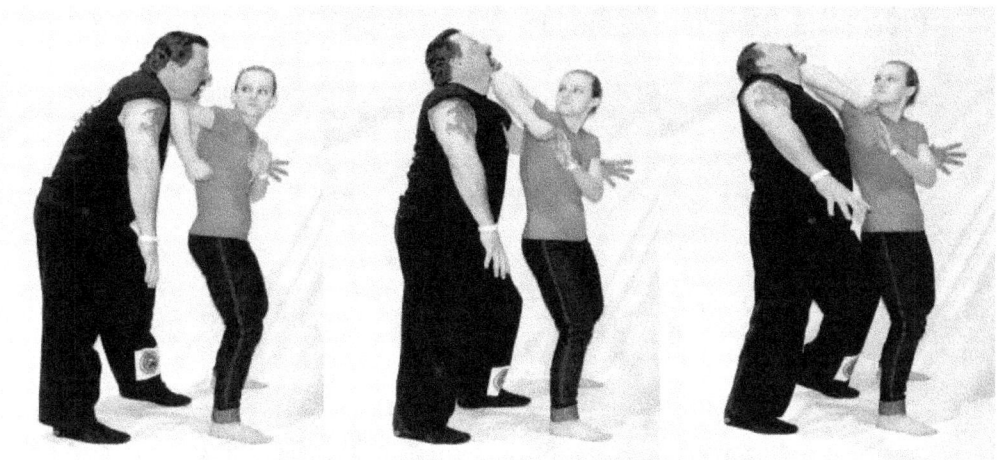

Immediately drive your elbow up under the attacker's chin into his throat, as hard and as high as you can, as if you're picking up a heavy suitcase.

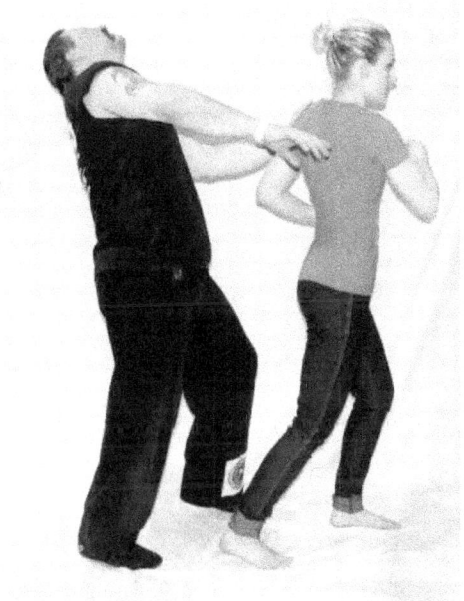

You can then escape quickly.

Note: You can mule kick the attacker in the groin again, as you escape the attack. The mule kick is done by kicking your heel back behind you and into the target.

Recap of the "Going on Vacation" technique:

1) Reach forward like you're grabbing your doorknob.

2) Pull the doorknob back as hard as you can.

3) Reach down for your luggage.

4) Pick up your luggage as high as you can.

Technique #10: "The Windmill"

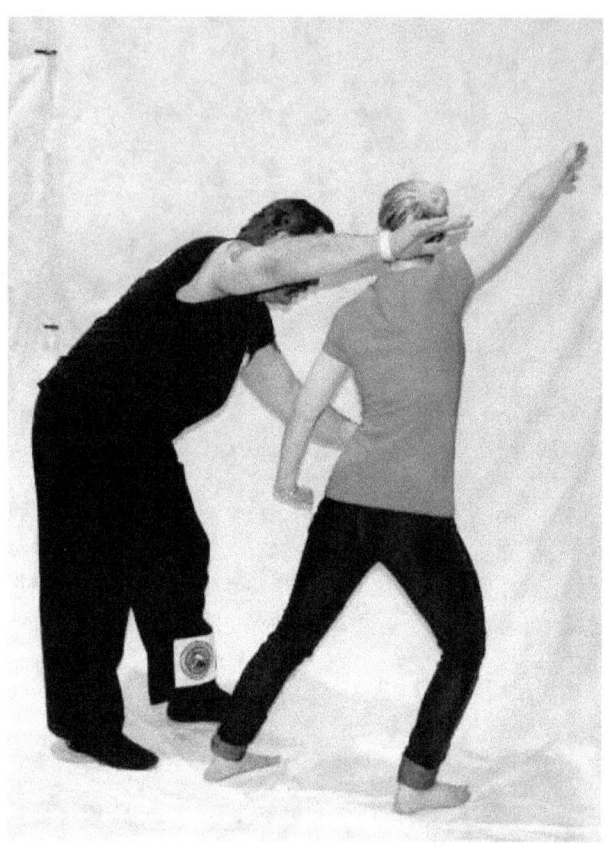

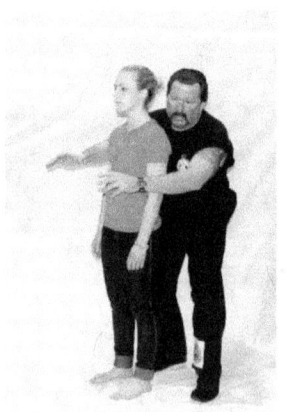 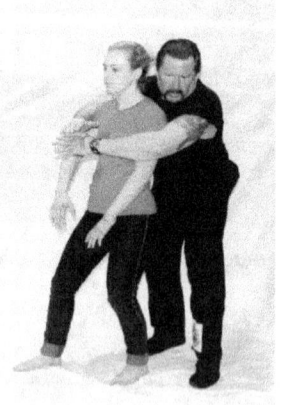 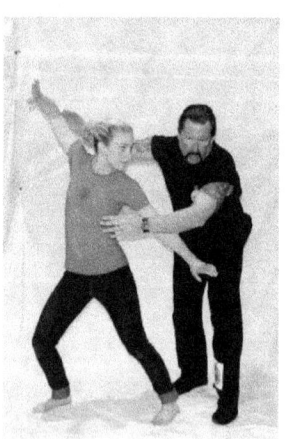

As the attacker is putting his arms around you, bend your knees slightly to lower your center of gravity. Keeping your arm straight, throw your right arm up towards your ear as hard as you can. While you are doing this, drop the other arm lower towards your own body.

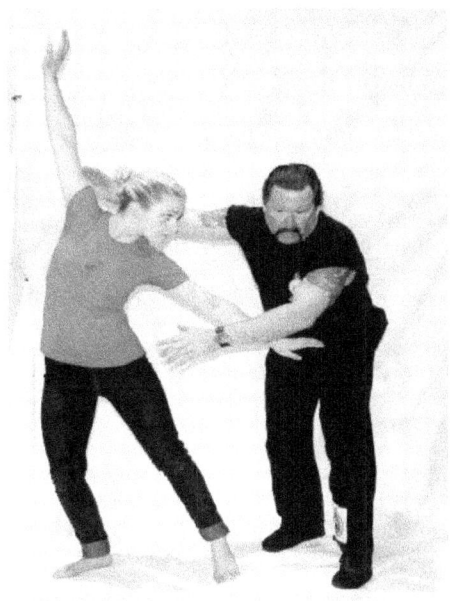 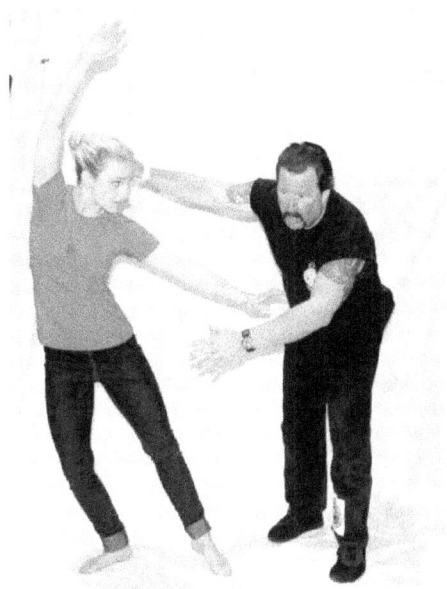

Spin out and around, rotating your body towards the attacker. This spin will loosen the attacker's grip and allow you to escape.

Note: This technique is effective when the attacker already has his arms around you or is attempting to bear hug you.

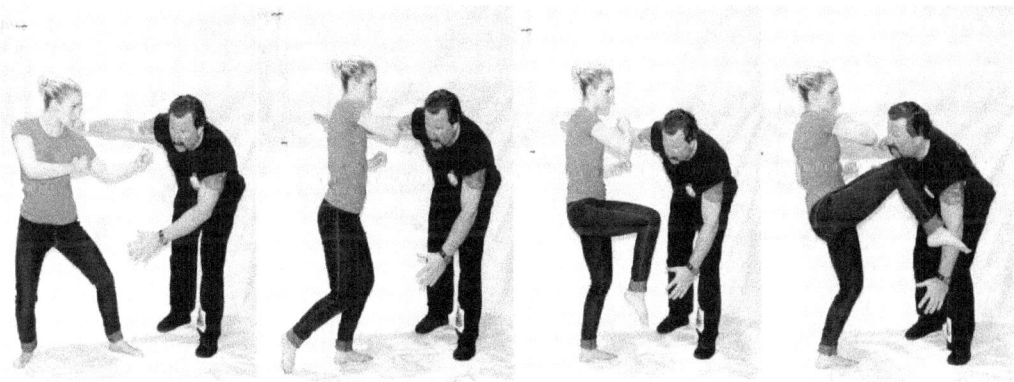

You are now positioned to drive your knee into the attacker's face. (The chin or the nose may be the most effective targets for the knee strike)

You are now set up for an elbow strike to the attacker's face. Step in towards the attacker and drive your elbow directly into his face as hard as you can. (The jaw, chin, nose, ear, or behind the ear are most effective targets for the elbow strike.)

Technique #11: Multiple Strike Series 4 (Duck/Punch/Knee Strike)

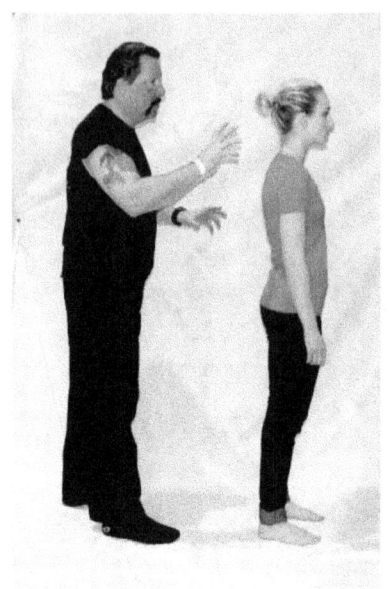 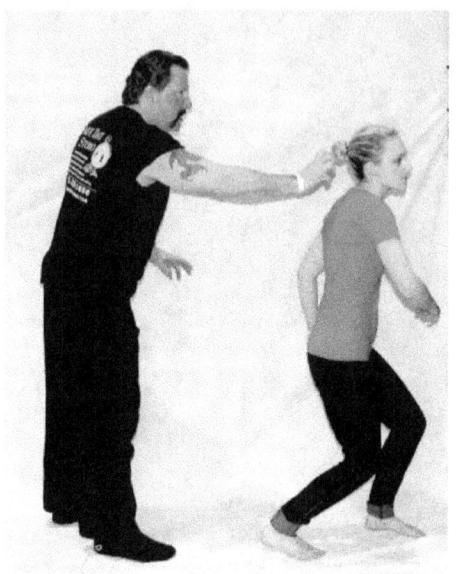

Attacker approaches from behind attempting to grab your hair

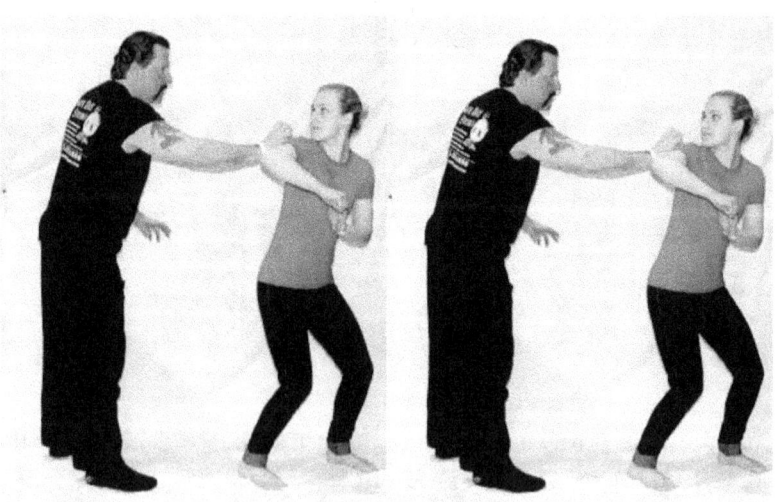

As you feel the attacker attempt to grab your hair, duck slightly to avoid having the attacker get a good grip on your hair. Then step forward with your left foot and start to swing your body around to the right towards your attacker (clockwise).

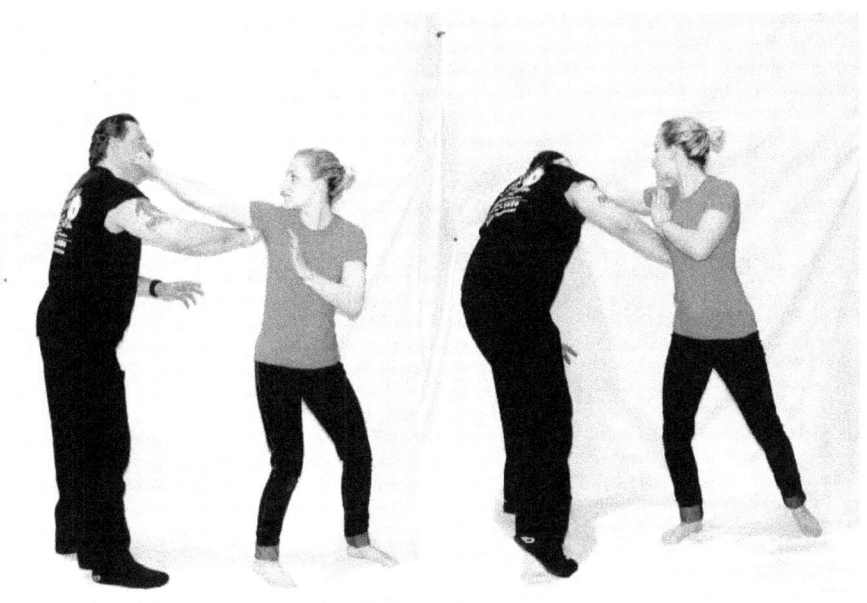

Strike the attacker's face with your fist as hard as you can.

Drive your fist into the attacker's jaw. There is a pressure point on the jaw bone that can knock out the attacker. This spot is located on the jawbone directly below the outer edge of the mouth.

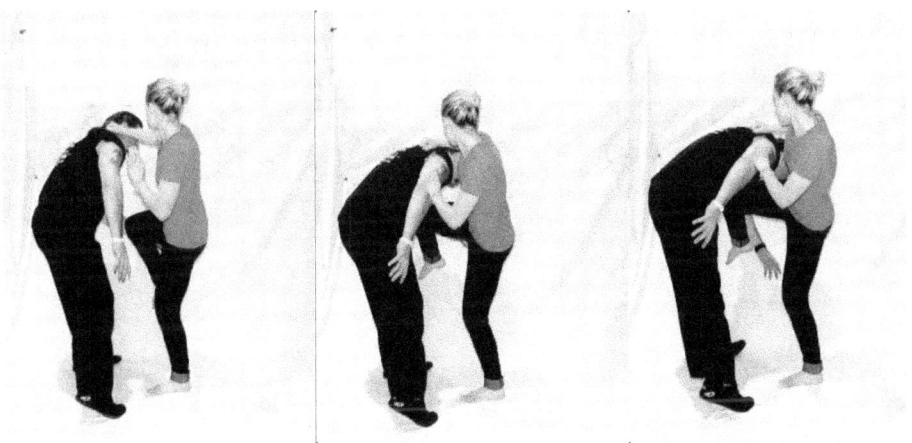

You can now pull the attacker's head down and drive your knee into the attacker's body or face. You can strike the solar plexus (center of chest), neck or face region. These regions are effective targets to strike and may do the most damage.

CHAPTER TWO TIPS:

- Don't hesitate to ask for an escort from a public safety officer or another trusted individual if you feel uneasy walking to your car from a restaurant, bar or mall.

- Move your cell phone from your purse to your front pocket or somewhere hidden from an attacker. That way you will have easy access to your phone and you will still have it with you if your handbag is taken.

- If you think you're being followed, try to confirm if you are. While observing the possible threat, change direction and/or stop walking. If the person you think is following you does the same, immediately seek safety in a public place or prepare for self-defense.

- Follow these tips on how to wear your hair:

  o **Worst option** – The **ponytail**

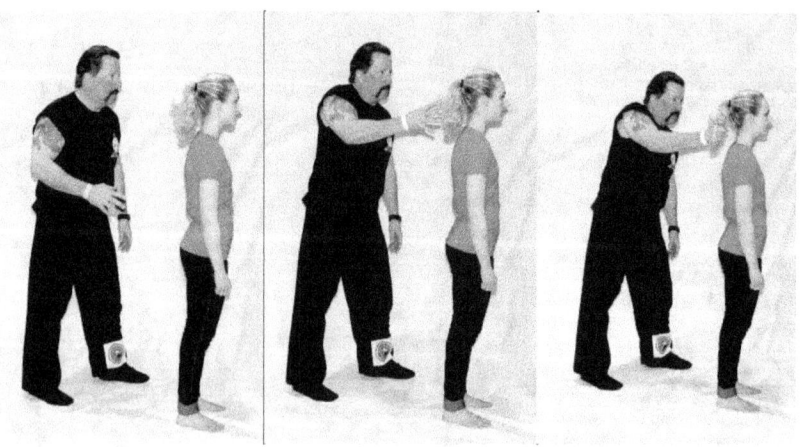

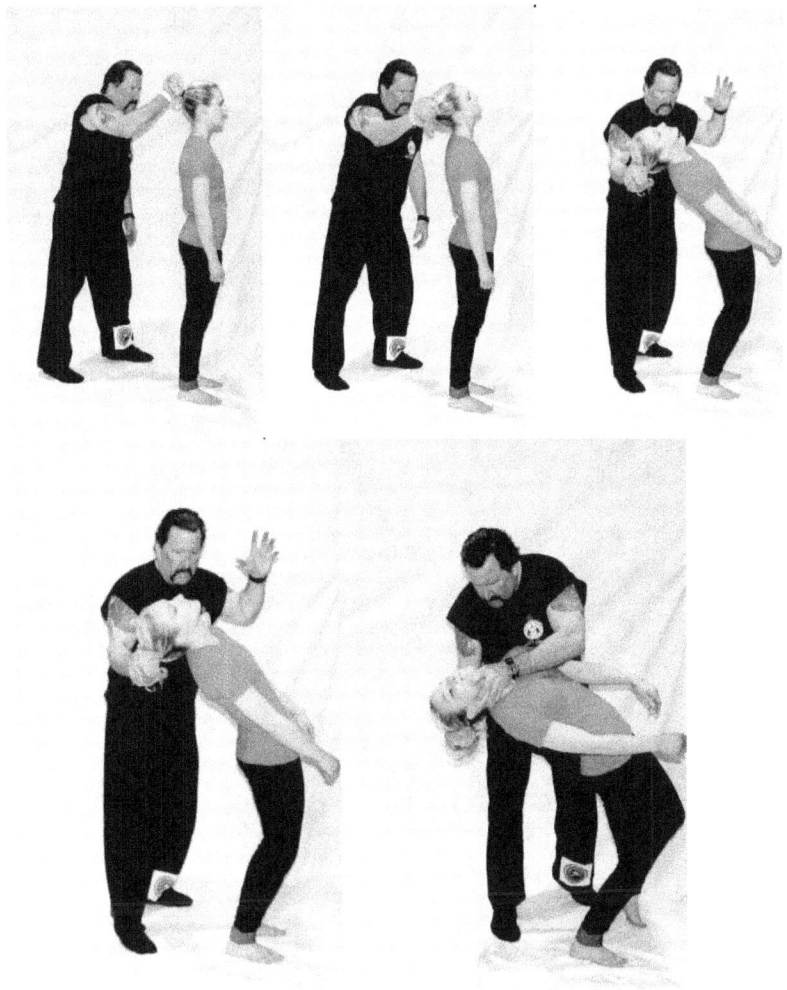

The attacker can come up behind you grabbing the ponytail like a handle. If the hair is long enough, an attacker can wrap his hand around it. When your hair is pulled together in a ponytail, you go where your hair goes! The attacker can easily pull you to the ground. Most of the time your head will be the first thing that hits the ground.

Note: You can always fix your hair when you get where you're going. Follow these tips!

- o **Better option** – Wear your hair **down and loose**. The attacker may get some hair, but you're more likely to be able to pull away. You may lose some hair and your head will be sore, but you'll be alive.

- o **Best option** – Wear your hair up in a **tight bun or up-do**. This makes it very difficult to grab and manipulate. This may discourage an attacker.

    Note: If you insist on wearing a ponytail, at least tuck it into the back of your shirt/jacket. While this option is better, it is still dangerous.

Michael E. Andrus

CHAPTER 3

KEEP BREATHING: DEFENDING AGAINST THE CHOKE

Quick, effective techniques to protect against a rear choke

Scenario: You are away on a business trip, and are eager to take your early morning run in a different city. The sights are interesting, and you are enjoying the relative solitude of a run at dusk. All of a sudden you sense a presence behind you. What do you do?

Rear Choke Defense

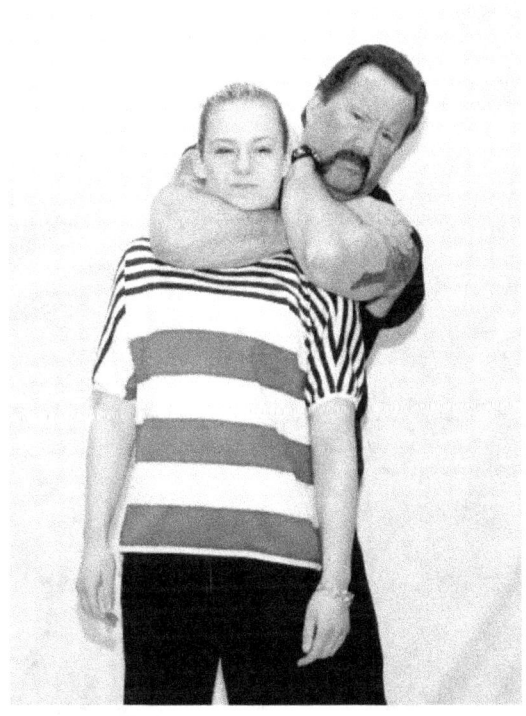

Technique #12: "Neck Guard"

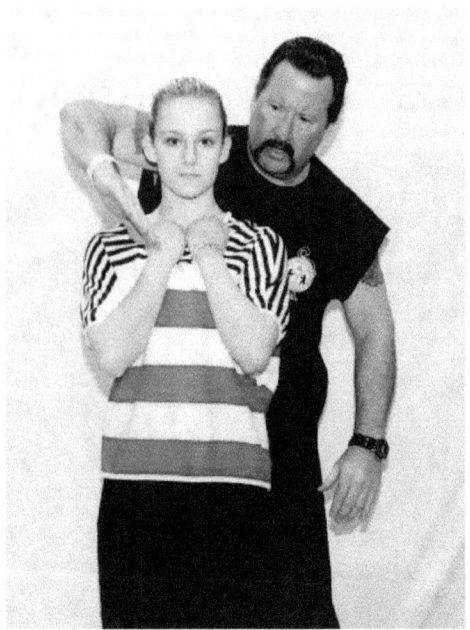

Attacker approaches from the rear.

Grab your shirt material tight with both hands under your neck.

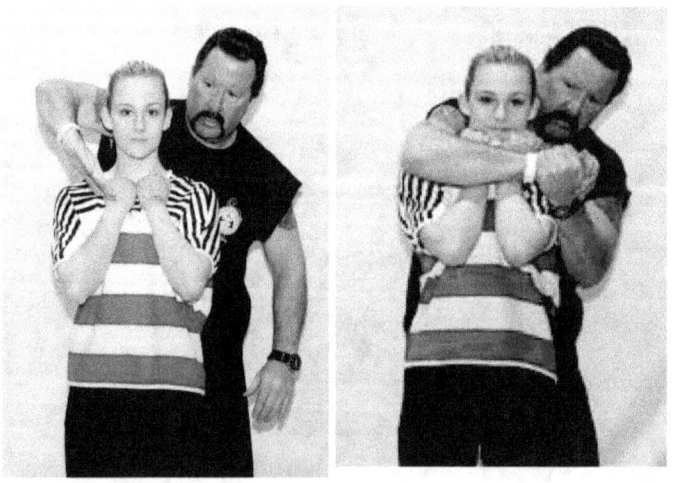

Pull up with both hands, pressing them firmly against your chin. Continue to keep your hands tight to your chin (The pressure of the attackers arms may hurt but you won't get choked out!) Kick backwards towards attacker's knee caps and shins. You can also sharply rake your heel down the front of the attacker's shins and stomp on the top part of his foot.

Option: You may also be able to duck out of this choke attempt.

Technique #13: "Duck Under"

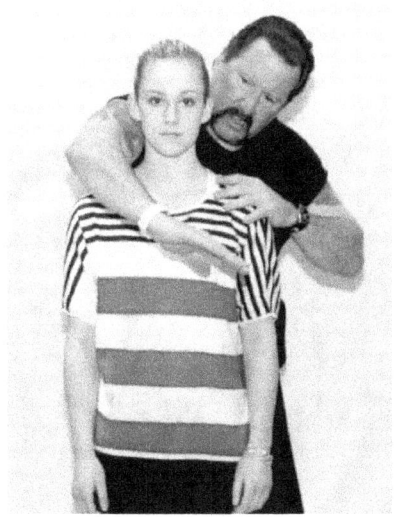

Attacker approaches from the rear.

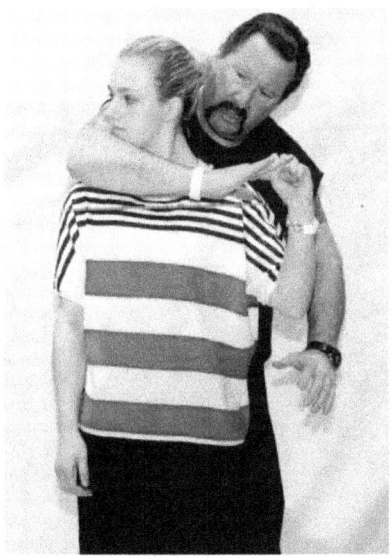

Drive your chin firmly into the inside crook of the attacker's bent arm, at the elbow. Keep your chin down, not allowing the attacker to get his arm up under your chin and around your neck. This technique will allow you to continue to breathe to complete your escape.

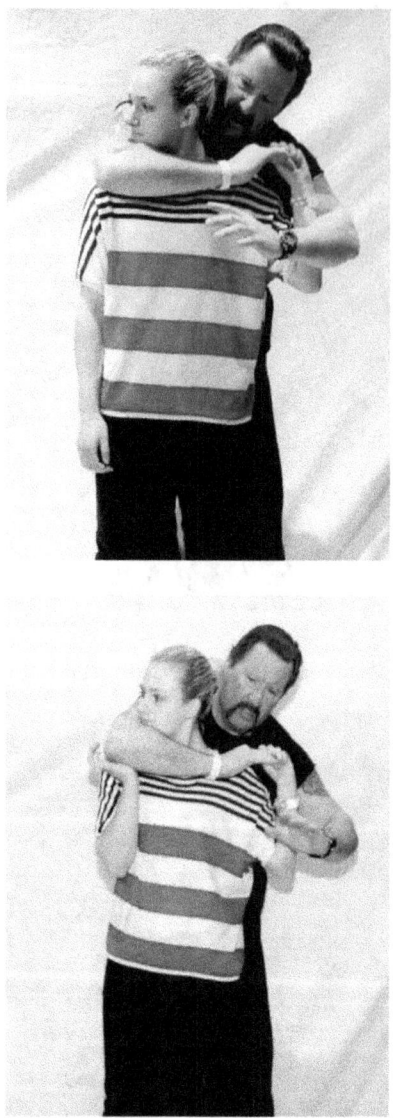

Reach for the attacker's fingers on the hand that is attempting to choke you.

Place your open available hand under the attacker's elbow (cupping it), while the other hand firmly grabs the fingers of the attacker.

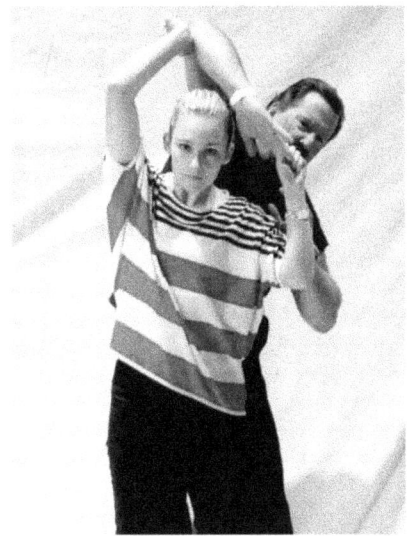

Push the attacker's elbow straight up as hard as you can while you quickly step forward. While pushing the elbow up and back behind you, continue to hold the fingers of the attacker with your other hand.

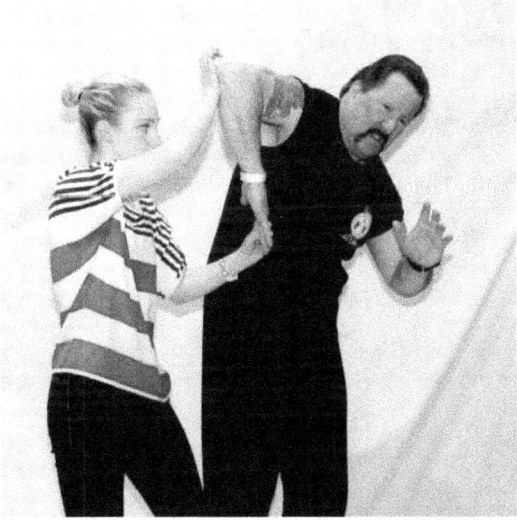

Step back and under the attacker's elbow. Keep constant pressure on the elbow and fingers. Bend the fingers of the attacker back as far and as hard as you can.

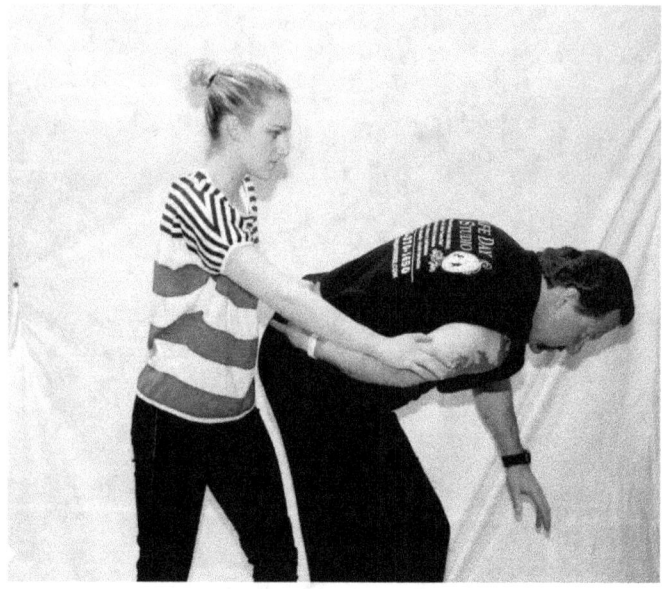

Push the attacker's elbow forward and down. Push the attacker forward as hard as you can.

You can now escape by running or kicking the attacker behind the knee or kick him in the groin from behind.

Technique #14: "Cobra Hand"

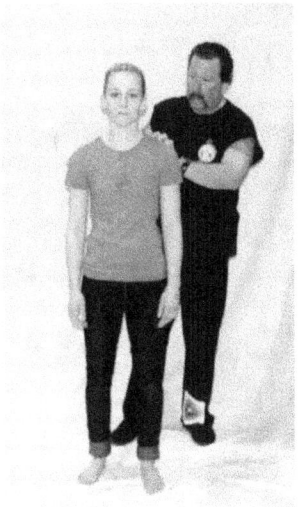

Attacker approaches from behind you.

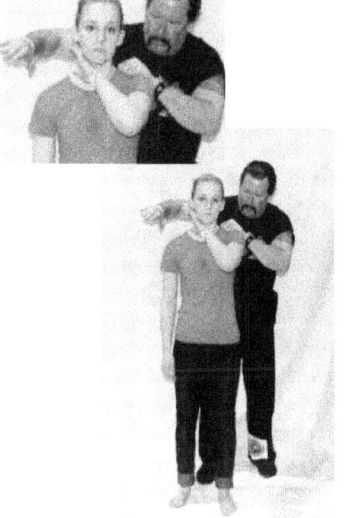

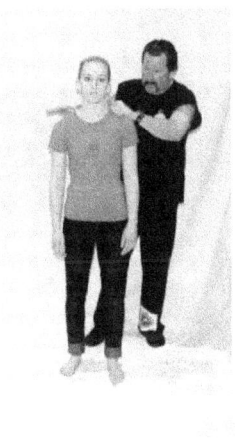

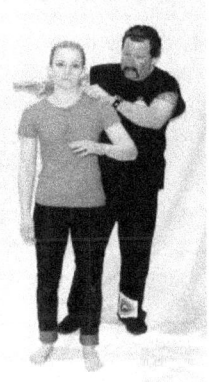

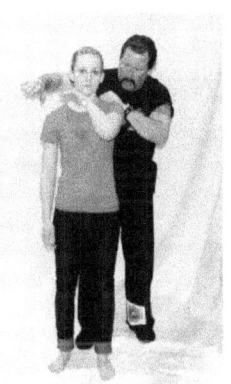

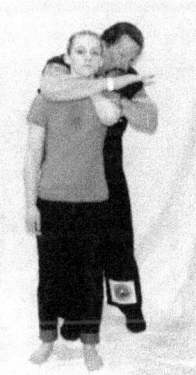

As you feel someone behind you, immediately bring your hand up in front of your neck (keep your hand open). Angle your hand out and away from your face and body. This creates a hook to catch the attacker's arm or hand as he attempts to wrap it around your neck. This protects you from being choked.

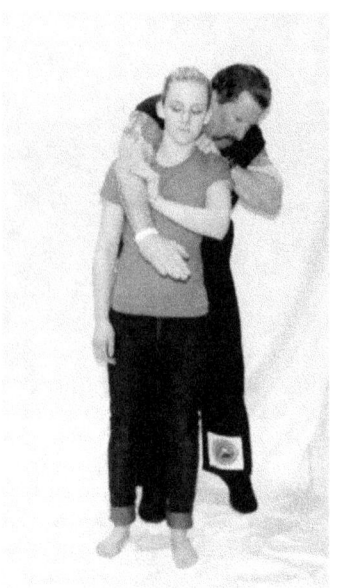

This hand position allows you to push the attacker's arm down and away from you.

Note: Once you are free from the choking hand you can use your heel to kick the attacker's leg while escaping and/or thrust your elbow into the attacker's ribs or solar plexus (center of the chest)

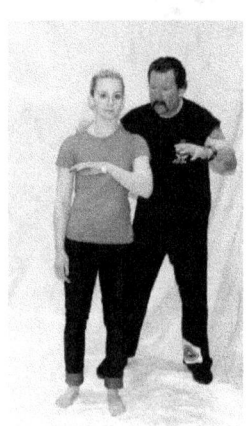
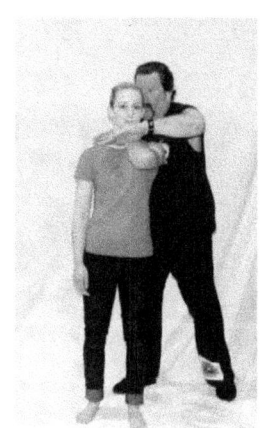
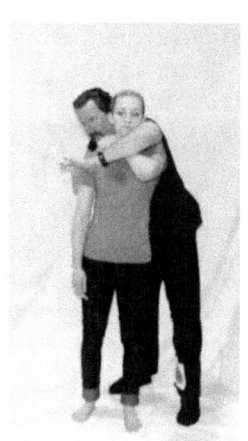

This technique is effective regardless of which hand the attacker is using.

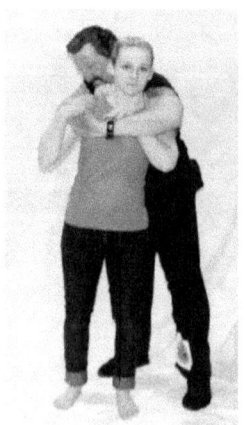
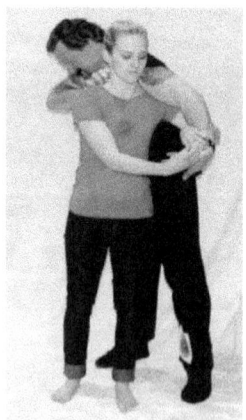

Grab the attacker's fingers on the choking hand and bend them back as far as you can and as hard as you can.

CHAPTER THREE TIPS:

- Exercise with another person or in a group whenever possible.

- Do not jog outside when it is dark or in an unfamiliar area EVER.

- Do not run in or past secluded areas.

- ALWAYS take your cell phone with you wherever you go. Your phone is your emergency lifeline.

- Leave an updated "flight plan" in your hotel room that details where you will be at all times. Having a detailed description of your daily activities at home is just as important.

- When using public transportation, research your route, including fare and timetables prior to traveling. Do not wait until you arrive at the terminal to ask others for travel information.

- Only use public transportation that is clearly marked as such. Never accept a ride from a "for-hire" driver unless you can verify proper identification.

- Remember, no ponytails!

Michael E. Andrus

CHAPTER 4

PRACTICE MAKES PERFECT: ARM GRAB DEFENSE

Quick, effective techniques to protect against a wrist or arm grab

Scenario: You are walking home from your regular bus stop after a long day at work. Since this is a route you have traveled many times, you listen to your iPod and zone out. Suddenly, a man walking past you grabs you by the arm. What do you do?

Wrist or arm grab defense
Technique #15: "The Iron"

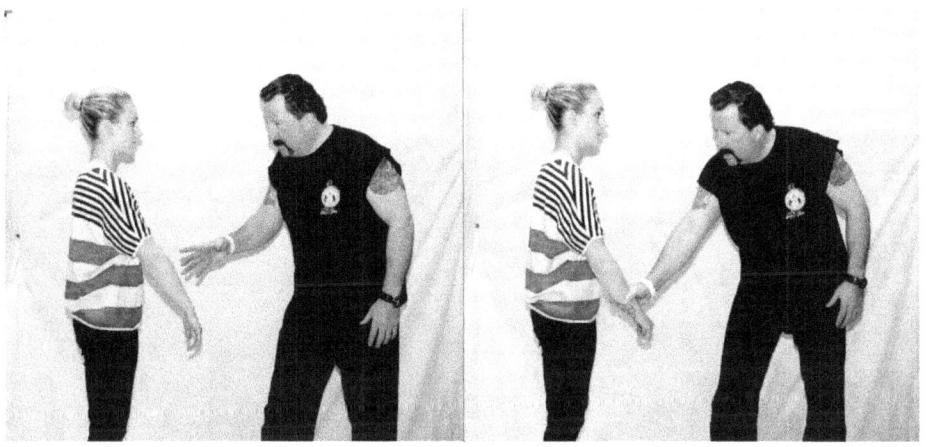

The attacker reaches and grabs your wrist and starts to pull you in.

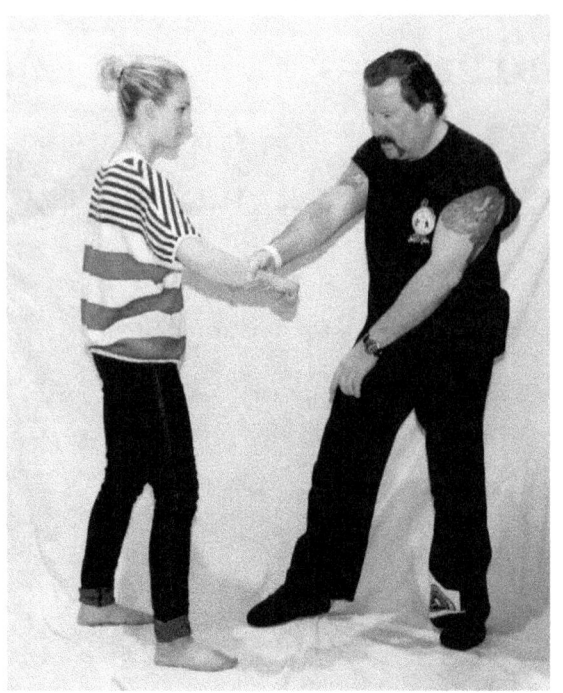

Step forward with your foot that is on the same side as the hand that is being grabbed. (e.g., step forward with your right foot if your right hand is being grabbed)

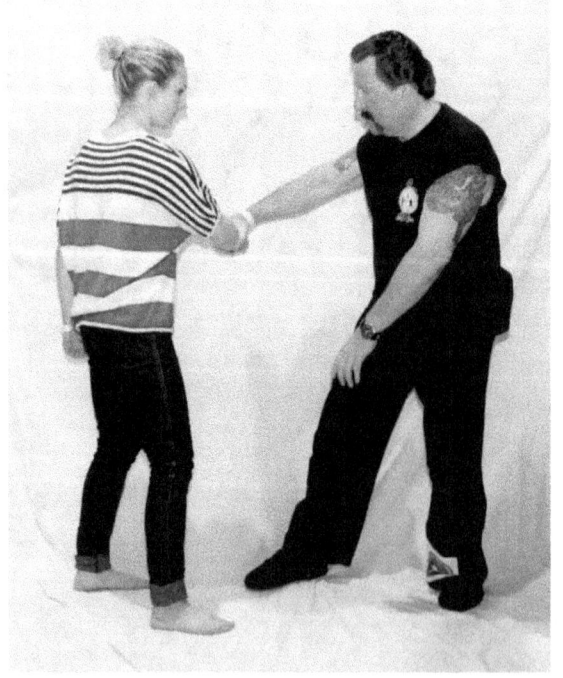

Move your hand firmly from right to left, parallel to the ground as if you were ironing across the front of your body.

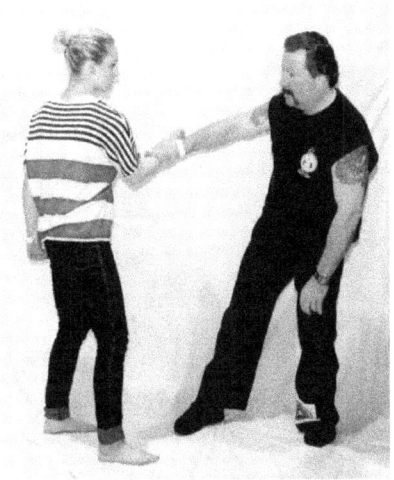 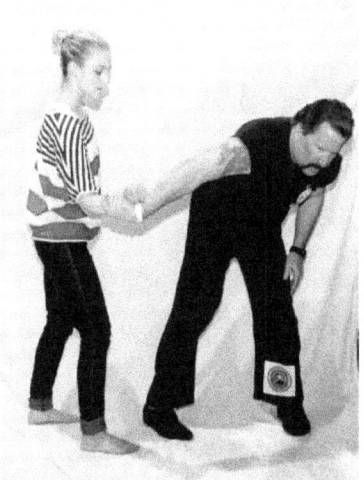

Then, flip your wrist over (upside down) and come back with your hand moving it firmly left to right. This motion will invert the attacker's hand and body position. (You are now ironing upside down and back the other direction)

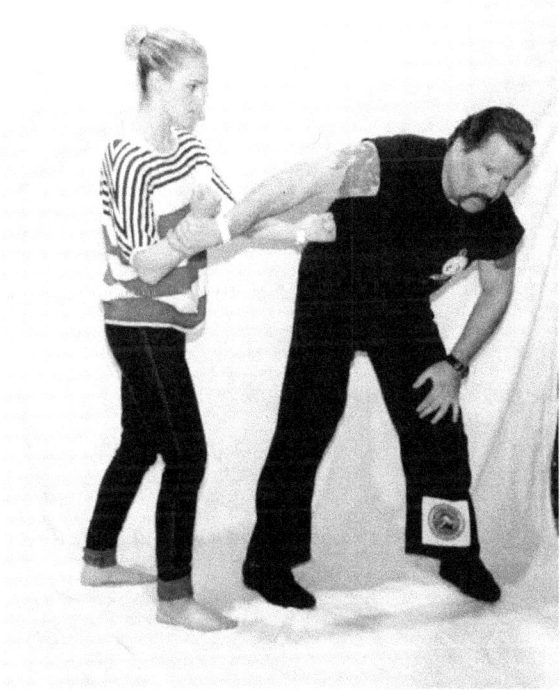

The attacker's rib cage is now exposed for multiple punches.

Continue to punch the attacker's ribs as many times and as hard as you can. Keep your hand in a fist upside down, which will enable your punch to strike an individual rib on the attacker. This hand position may increase your chances of breaking one or several of the attacker's ribs.

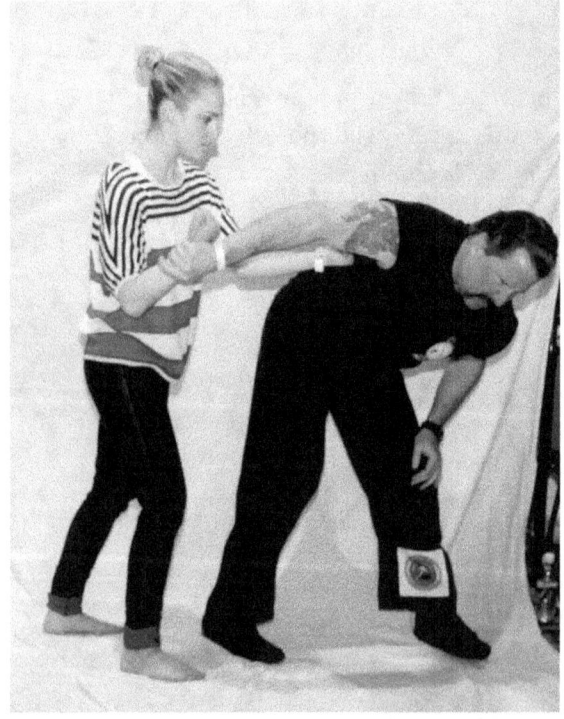

Note: It is difficult to breathe or run with broken ribs. An attacker may be less likely to run after you if he has broken or bruised ribs.

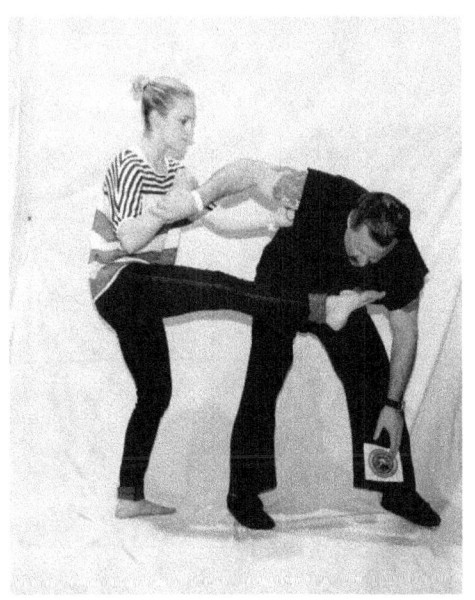 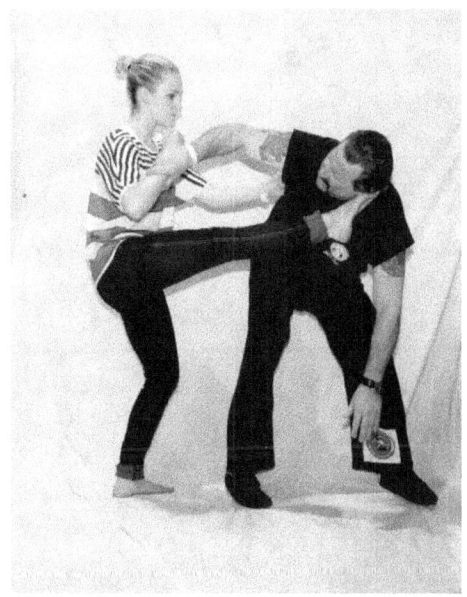

You can kick the attacker in the face or head region after or during rib punches. Kick as hard as you can to the face to break the nose or to the side of the head to damage the ear and neck.

Opposite angle showing the same technique

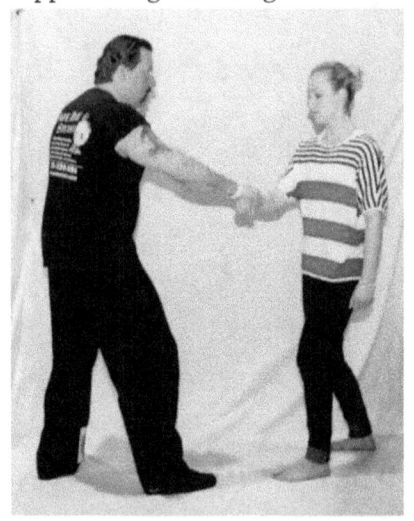
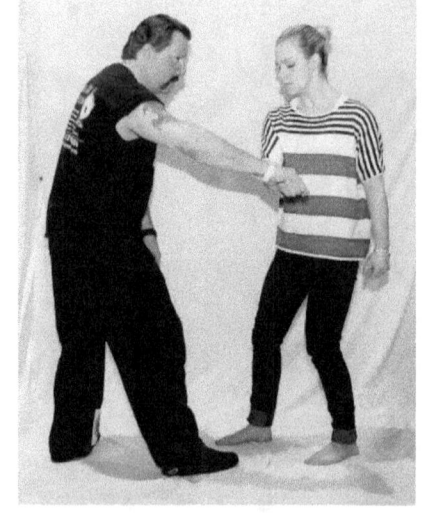

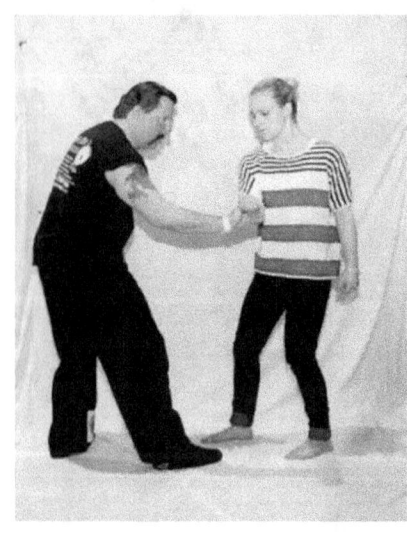
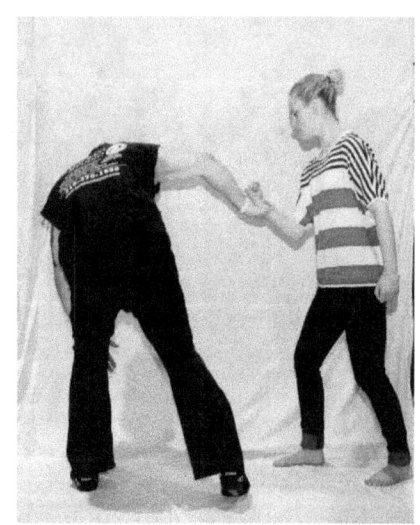

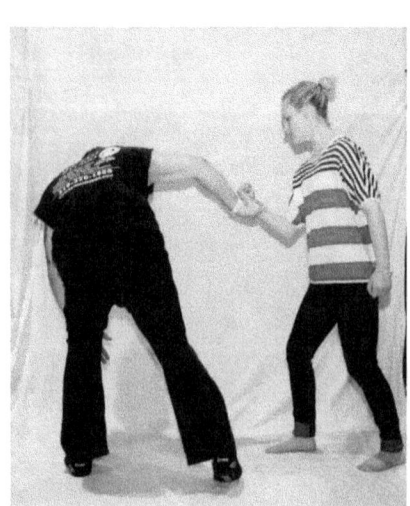
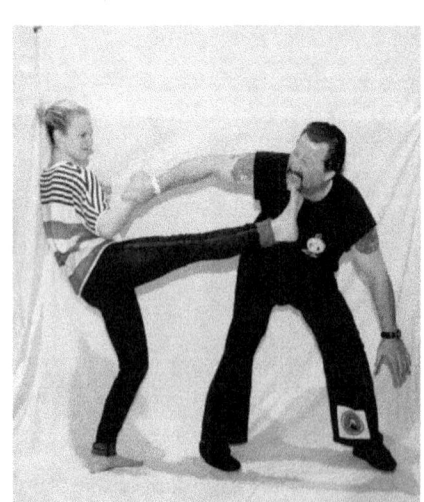

CHAPTER FOUR TIPS:

- When taking public transportation or walking, don't dress to attract unwanted attention. Short skirts and low necklines may do just that. Wear practical shoes while in transit. You can always remove extra clothing or change your shoes when you get to where you're going.

- Do not wear a tight cross-body bag that you can't quickly remove. Do not wear a backpack that has a handle on the back. If you wear a backpack, keep it loose enough that you can free your arms if it is pulled.

- Tell someone where you are going and what time you'll be returning.

- Carry your purse in your non-dominant hand to keep your dominant hand free to protect you. Defending yourself with your dominant hand allows a quicker and more accurate defense.

- In public, do not wear both ear buds, so you can stay alert to sounds around you.

- Practice these techniques until they become second nature.

CHAPTER 5

ADDITIONAL SAFETY TIPS

- Charge your cell phone in your bedroom at home, not in the kitchen. You want to have immediate access in case of an emergency.

- If you hear a dog barking outside your home, check it out. It may be something—dogs bark for a reason!

- If you feel you must hide, do not hide in a crouched position. You cannot kick, punch or run from that position. Also don't hide under your bed. You can't protect yourself from there either.

- Keep weapons hidden around the house that you have been trained to use, such as edged weapons, sticks, pepper spray, etc.

- If you have an alarm on your car keychain, keep it close to you when you're sleeping. That way, if you feel you are in danger, you can use your car alarm to alert neighbors.

- If you dial 911, remember to calmly and quickly tell them where you are in as much detail as possible. Also, as calmly and quickly as possible, let them know the nature of your problem. (i.e. "I'm being followed", "There's a stranger in my house," "I have been threatened," etc.).

- Make sure you carry your cell phone or weapon on your person. Nothing in your purse can be effective if it is taken away.

- If you choose to carry pepper spray, or any weapon, get trained on how to use it first. Otherwise, you may only be providing your attacker with a weapon to use against you.

- If you are walking to your car in a parking garage, don't walk close to the columns. Someone could easily be hiding behind them, and you won't see them until it's too late!

- If someone asks for help while you are in your car, keep your doors locked and your windows up. You can hear them through the window. If you determine the emergency to be valid, you can call 911 for help.

- Practice deep breathing—in through your nose and out through your mouth. Deep breathing can keep you calm and keep oxygen going to your lungs and brain, which is necessary to think and act fast.

- Always look in front, to the sides and behind you, wherever you are!

- Do not stand in a public place with your legs crossed. You have no balance in that position. Instead, get used to standing in a strong stance so that if you were pushed, pulled or shoved you won't lose your balance.

- Confuse your attacker by speaking slowly and softly. Doing so may trick the attacker into moving his face closer to you so you can attack it!

- Use every weapon you have! Your head, shoulders, elbows, fists, fingers, fingernails, knees and feet are weapons.

- The rules are; there are no rules! Use every means you have to hurt your attacker and survive.

- If you find yourself at gun point and you can escape, run in a zig-zag pattern away from the attacker. The odds of your attacker missing you are quadrupled!

- If you can escape, do it. If you can't escape, fight. If you must fight, win! DON'T BE A VICTIM!

The techniques in this book may give you an opportunity to save your life or the life of a loved one. Make a commitment to yourself to understand and practice these techniques on a regular basis. The ability to apply what you learn is the key to survival.

REMEMBER: Stay in the moment and have a Safe Day!